Breastfeeding:

Conditions and Diseases

A Reference Guide

Breastfeeding:

Conditions and Diseases

A Reference Guide

First Edition

Anne Merewood, MA, IBCLC
Director of Lactation Services
The Breastfeeding Center
Boston Medical Center

Barbara L. Philipp, MD, IBCLC
Assistant Professor of Pediatrics
Boston University School of Medicine
Chief, Division of Pediatric Ambulatory Services
Medical Director, The Breastfeeding Center
Boston Medical Center

Pharmasoft Publishing
Breastfeeding: Conditions and Diseases

A Reference Guide

First Edition

© Copyright 2001

Pharmasoft Publishing

http://iBreastfeeding.com

(806)-376-9900
(800)-378-1317

DISCLAIMER

ISBN   0-9636219-5-5

2

For Gregory, Alexi, Dimitri, and Mike
Anne Merewood

❦

For Vince, Jessie, Nick and Abby

Bobbi Philipp

3

Acknowledgements

The authors would like to thank colleagues Kim Barbas, BSN, IBCLC, and Liz Brown, MD for their clinical advice during the compellation of this manuscript, and Tom Hale, PhD for his editorial insights.

The authors would also like to thank Barry Zuckerman, MD for his powerful support and vision; Howard Bauchner, MD for his friendship and academic support; and Bob Vinci, MD for his unparalleled commitment to the breastfeeding cause. We would also like to thank Esther Gerendas, PNP, IBCLC because she is always there with us, working for our breastfeeding families at Boston Medical Center.

Anne Merewood
Bobbi Philipp

Contents

Contents

Contents

Introduction

As health care professionals working daily with breastfeeding women at Boston Medical Center (BMC), a Baby-Friendly™, inner city hospital with 1800 births per year, we receive frequent requests for information from mothers and fellow clinicians, on medical issues surrounding lactation. *Breastfeeding: Conditions and Diseases* is intended as a reference guide for our health care colleagues: physicians, nurses, lactation consultants, midwives, physicians' assistants, nurse practitioners, and breastfeeding counselors – health care staff at all levels who are working as we are to assist and support breastfeeding women.

This book addresses a wide spectrum of common and less common maternal and infant conditions and diseases, and in each case seeks to answer the question: Can the mother or baby breastfeed? In the vast majority of instances, the answer is yes. Using evidence based-research, the book explains why breastfeeding is, in most cases, appropriate; provides information on any necessary precautions; offers tips for breastfeeding in challenging situations, and addresses issues associated with medications and breastmilk.

According to the American Academy of Pediatrics, breastfeeding is "the optimal form of nutrition for all infants." According to the United States Surgeon General, breastfeeding is the "ideal method of feeding and nurturing infants", and a national health priority. According to Healthy People 2010, the US national goal is for 75% of women to initiate breastfeeding, 50% of women to breastfeed until six months, and 25% of women to breastfeed their children until one year of age. Breastfeeding goals for Healthy People 2000 were not met. With approximately 64% of US mothers now initiating breastfeeding, 20% breastfeeding at six months, and 16% breastfeeding at one year, objectives for 2010 are far from assured.

Clinicians who work with women and children share a mutual obligation to encourage and promote breastfeeding initiation and duration through the provision of appropriate, consistent advice for breastfeeding mothers. We hope that this book will assist our fellow health care professionals in offering accurate, research-based information on lactation, and will serve as a resource to ensure that greater numbers of women ultimately succeed in their decision to provide the healthiest start possible for their children.

Anne Merewood
Barbara Philipp

Acrodermatitis enteropathica

Summary

Breastfeeding should be strongly encouraged for infants with acrodermatitis enteropathica.

Definition/cause

Acrodermatitis enteropathica is an autosomal recessive disorder in which patients suffer from a malabsorption of zinc from the gastrointestinal tract. Onset can be as early as three weeks of life, but is delayed in breastfeeding infants and may not become apparent until the child is weaned from breastmilk. The age of onset therefore varies, but the average is around nine months.[1]

Signs and symptoms

The disease is characterized by a triad of dermatitis, diarrhea and alopecia. It begins with a rash located around body orifices such as the mouth, nose, eyes, ears, and perineum. The lesions begin as vesicles, bullae and pustules that denude and become dry, scaly, and crusted with a well-defined border. If untreated, the disease progresses and the eczematoid rash is located symmetrically on the buttocks, cheeks, knees and elbows, and on the fingers and toes. The hair acquires a reddish tint, alopecia occurs, and eye abnormalities such as photophobia, conjunctivitis, blepharitis and corneal dystrophy can occur. Other symptoms include chronic diarrhea, stomatitis and glossitis (causing drooling), nail dystrophy, growth retardation, irritable mental status, apathy, listlessness, and secondary bacterial or candidal infections The wide range of findings relate to zinc's role in white blood cell activity, and copper, protein, essential fatty acid and prostaglandin metabolic pathways.

Diagnosis is made by the characteristic clinical findings and abnormal serum zinc levels.

Treatment

Exclusive breastfeeding, which may involve increasing the maternal milk supply or relactation, is an effective treatment for the infant under six months of age. For formula-fed infants and older patients, treatment is the daily, oral administration of zinc and continual

13

monitoring of zinc levels. With treatment, there is rapid healing of skin lesions and improvement of the diarrhea and other symptoms.

Breastfeeding and acrodermatitis enteropathica

Breastfeeding is protective and delays the onset of this illness. Although breastmilk contains less zinc than cow's milk, the zinc in human milk forms a complex with prostaglandin E and is better absorbed.[2]

The mother of an infant with acrodermatitis enteropathica should be made aware that the longer she breastfeeds, the less zinc supplementation the infant will need. If she is primarily breastfeeding, but offering formula supplements, she may be able to increase her milk supply by more frequent nursing, or by using an electric breast pump (see Low milk supply), and breastfeed her infant exclusively. Relactation, which involves recreating the milk supply through regular use of a breast pump (see Adoptive nursing) and by putting the infant to breast as frequently as possible, is another option. Despite the protective effects of breastfeeding, there is no added benefit to be had by maternal zinc supplementation, because zinc levels in milk are independent of maternal intake.

Food for thought

- Danbolt and Closs described and named the disease in 1942, hence the alternative name of Danbolt-Closs syndrome. However, the disease continued to baffle scientists until 1973 when Moynahan discovered the relationship with zinc malabsorption.
- If a chronic diaper rash refuses to resolve, and common causes such as candidal infection and bacterial superinfection have been ruled out, the clinician should consider psoriasis and acrodermatitis enteropathica.

References

1. Hurwitz S. *Clinical Pediatric Dermatology:A Textbook of Skin Disorders of Childhood and Adolesence.* Philadelphia:WB Saunders;1981:31-33
2. Lawrence RA, Lawrence RM. *Breastfeeding: A Guide for the Medical Profession.* 5th ed. St Louis:Mosby;1999:476-77.

Acute gastroenteritis

Summary
If the infant has an acute episode of gastroenteritis, the mother should be encouraged to continue breastfeeding. If the mother has acute gastroenteritis, she can continue to breastfeed. Hundreds of studies indicate that breastfeeding significantly reduces the risk of developing acute gastroenteritis in infants and young children worldwide.

Definition/cause
Acute gastroenteritis can be caused by many different infectious agents. Rotavirus is a common viral cause; implicated bacteria can include *salmonella, shigella, Campylobacter jejuni, Clostridium difficile, Yersinia enterocolitica,* and *Escherichia coli.* Parasites such as *giardia lamblia,* and *cryptosporidium* can also be responsible. The infection injures intestinal epithelial cells, making the necessary enzymes unavailable for digestion.

Worldwide, diarrhea causes over 3,000,000 deaths per year in children under five years of age.[1] Many deaths occur in areas where the causative agents of gastroenteritis thrive and propagate due to poor sanitation. In these conditions, not breastfeeding increases the cumulative risk of infection, gastroenteritis, diarrhea, dehydration and death because the anti-infective properties of colostrum and breastmilk are not present in formula, sterilization is not available, and there is a lack of clean water for making up formula or for washing feeding implements. Where families are poor and formula is expensive, bottle-fed babies risk receiving over-diluted formula and inadequate nutritional substitutes such as unpasteurized ('raw') cow's or goat's milk, rice water, sugar water, juice, and water.

The protective effects of breastmilk against diarrhea are not limited to underdeveloped nations. Scariati[26] found that when compared with exclusively breastfed infants, exclusively formula-fed infants in the U.S. had an 80% increased risk of developing diarrhea.

Signs and symptoms
Acute gastroenteritis is associated with diarrhea and vomiting, with or without fever. Diarrhea is defined as passing excessive stool with

increased water content. The child may be fussy, afebrile or have low grade fever, and suffer abdominal pain. Loose stools may escape the diaper and run down the leg; sometimes the stool contains mucous strands or bloody streaks. If the diarrhea continues or the infant's condition worsens, the parents should contact a clinician. The prime concern is to prevent dehydration due to excessive water loss.

Treatment

Adults with acute gastroenteritis should drink plenty of fluids to remain hydrated, and the breastfeeding infant should continue to breastfeed. If the infant becomes dehydrated, IV fluids or oral rehydration solutions may also be needed. If the causative agent is bacterial, antibiotics may be prescribed as indicated.

Acute gastroenteritis and breastfeeding
Protective effects

Studies on infant mortality in two urban areas of southern Brazil found that bottle-fed infants had a 14.2 times higher risk of death than their exclusively breastfed peers.[2] Another study, in a Brazilian shanty town, examined persistent diarrhea (episodes lasting more than 14 days) in children under three, and found that exclusively breastfed children had 8-fold lower diarrhea rates than formula-fed children. The main causes of persistent diarrhea were *cryptosporidium parvum, giardia lamblia*, enteric adenoviruses, and enterotoxigenic *Escherichia coli*.[3] Studies consistently show that breastfeeding prevents or decreases the severity of diarrheal episodes and associated morbidity.[1, 4-9] One meta-analysis of 35 studies from 14 countries showed a 3.5-4.9 fold higher risk of diarrhea among bottle fed infants than breastfed infants in the first six months of life.[5]

Exclusive breastfeeding, early initiation of breastfeeding, and duration of breastfeeding are all associated with decreased gastroenteritis. One study found that formula-fed infants had 4.7-16.8 times more diarrhea than exclusively breastfed infants.[10] Another showed that infants who began breastfeeding by day three of life had a 26% lower rate of diarrhea over the first six months of life than infants who began later: researchers hypothesized that this outcome was due to the protective effects of colostrum.[11]

Not all research focuses on developing nations. According to a study of over 8000 English children, breastfeeding was positively correlated with a decreased infant diarrhea and decreased morbidity in the United Kingdom in the 1990s.[12] Another study looked at the effect of breastfeeding on diarrhea among affluent USA families, and found that diarrhea was halved in the breastfed infants.[6] Additionally, a literature review disclosed a significant protective effect of breastfeeding on diarrheal episodes in both developed and non-developed nations.[4]

Reasons for the protective effects of breastmilk abound. Compared to the formula-fed infant, flora in the gut of the breastfed infant has more bifidobacteria and lactobacillus. Several components of human milk, including secretory IgA, oligosaccharides, glycolipids, glycoproteins and lactoferrins provide defense against specific enteric pathogens such as: *Campylobacter jejuni, Clostridium difficile, Escherichia coli, Giardia lamblia,* rotavirus, *Salmonella typhimurium, Shigella* and *Vibrio cholerae.*[13] In addition to transferring passive immunity, breastmilk may contain active anti-inflammatory agents.[14] Specific studies have found a protective effect of breastmilk against *Cryptosporidium parvum,*[15] *Escherichia coli,*[16,17] and rotavirus.[18]

Diarrhea in the breastfed baby

The normal stool from a breastfed infant is loose, bright yellow, chunky (like liquid mustard with cottage cheese lumps), and often passed with every feed. This may confuse parents who often think the frequent loose stool is diarrhea. Additional symptoms, such as crankiness and vomiting, can help make the diagnosis. The best solution is to continue breastfeeding, offer oral rehydration fluids as necessary, and watch the infant for signs of dehydration (see Dehydration).

Food for thought

- In 1991 UNICEF and the World Health Organization launched the Baby-Friendly Hospital Initiative (BFHI) in an attempt to decrease infant mortality and increase breastfeeding rates worldwide. To gain Baby-Friendly status, hospitals must meet specific criteria related to supporting and promoting breastfeeding as defined by the *Ten Steps to Successful Breastfeeding.* Currently, some 16,000 birthing sites internationally have received Baby-Friendly designation, and Baby-Friendly policies have successfully increased breastfeeding rates when put into practice.[19-26]

- Dubious marketing practices by various formula manufacturers, especially in third world countries, and images of dehydrated bottle-fed infants, led to an international boycott of Nestle in the 1970s, and the development of the WHO's International Code of Marketing of Breastmilk Substitutes.

References

1. Gracey M. Nutritional effects and management of diarrhoea in infancy. *Acta Paediatr Suppl* 1999;88(430):110-26.
2. Victora CG, Smith PG, Vaughan JP, Nobre LC, Lombardi C, Teixeira AM, et al. Evidence for protection by breast-feeding against infant deaths from infectious diseases in Brazil. *Lancet* 1987;2(8554):319-22.
3. Lima AA, Moore SR, Barboza MS, Jr., Soares AM, Schleupner MA, Newman RD, et al. Persistent diarrhea signals a critical period of increased diarrhea burdens and nutritional shortfalls: a prospective cohort study among children in northeastern Brazil. *J Infect Dis* 2000;181(5):1643-51.
4. Golding J, Emmett PM, Rogers IS. Gastroenteritis, diarrhoea and breast feeding. *Early Hum Dev* 1997;49 Suppl:S83-103.
5. Feachem RG, Koblinsky MA. Interventions for the control of diarrhoeal diseases among young children: promotion of breast-feeding. *Bull World Health Organ* 1984;62(2):271-91.
6. Dewey KG, Heinig MJ, Nommsen-Rivers LA. Differences in morbidity between breast-fed and formula-fed infants. *J Pediatr* 1995;126(5 Pt 1):696-702.
7. Beaudry M, Dufour R, Marcoux S. Relation between infant feeding and infections during the first six months of life. *J Pediatr* 1995;126(2):191-7.
8. Popkin BM, Adair L, Akin JS, Black R, Briscoe J, Flieger W. Breast-feeding and diarrheal morbidity. *Pediatrics* 1990;86(6):874-82.
9. Brown KH, Black RE, Lopez de Romana G, Creed de Kanashiro H. Infant-feeding practices and their relationship with diarrheal and other diseases in Huascar (Lima), Peru. *Pediatrics* 1989;83(1):31-40.
10. Howie PW, Forsyth JS, Ogston SA, Clark A, Florey CD. Protective effect of breast feeding against infection. *BMJ* 1990;300(6716):11-6.
11. Clemens J, Elyazeed RA, Rao M, Savarino S, Morsy BZ, Kim Y, et al. Early initiation of breastfeeding and the risk of infant diarrhea in rural Egypt. *Pediatrics* 1999;104(1):e3.
12. Baker D, Taylor H, Henderson J. Inequality in infant morbidity: causes and consequences in England in the 1990s. ALSPAC Study Team. Avon Longitudinal Study of Pregnancy and Childhood. *J Epidemiol Community Health* 1998;52(7):451-8.
13. Churchill RB, Pickering LK. The pros (many) and cons (a few) of breastfeeding. *Contemporary Pediatrics* 1998;15(12):108-119.

14. Hanson LA. Breastfeeding provides passive and likely long-lasting active immunity. *Ann Allergy Asthma Immunol* 1998;81(6):523-33; quiz 533-4, 537.
15. Bhattacharya MK, Teka T, Faruque AS, Fuchs GJ. Cryptosporidium infection in children in urban Bangladesh. *J Trop Pediatr* 1997;43(5):282-6.
16. Clemens JD, Rao MR, Chakraborty J, Yunus M, Ali M, Kay B, et al. Breastfeeding and the risk of life-threatening enterotoxigenic escherichia coli diarrhea in Bangladeshi infants and children. *Pediatrics* 1997;100(6):E2.
17. Long K, Vasquez-Garibay E, Mathewson J, de la Cabada J, DuPont H. The impact of infant feeding patterns on infection and diarrheal disease due to enterotoxigenic Escherichia coli. *Salud Publica Mex* 1999;41(4):263-70.
18. Naficy AB, Abu-Elyazeed R, Holmes JL, Rao MR, Savarino SJ, Kim Y, et al. Epidemiology of rotavirus diarrhea in Egyptian children and implications for disease control. *Am J Epidemiol* 1999;150(7):770-7.
19. Philipp BL, Merewood A, O'Brien S. US physicians and the promotion of breastfeeding: A Call for Action. *Pediatrics* 2001;107(3):584-588.
20. Merewood A, Philipp BL. Becoming Baby-Friendly: Overcoming the Issue of Accepting Free Formula. *Journal of Human Lactation* 2000;16(4):279-282.
21. Merewood A, Philipp BL. Implementing change: becoming Baby-Friendly in an inner city hospital. *Birth* 2001;28(1).
22. Saadeh R, Akre J. Ten steps to successful breastfeeding: a summary of the rationale and scientific evidence. *Birth* 1996;23(3):154-60.
23. Wright A, Rice S, Wells S. Changing hospital practices to increase the duration of breastfeeding. *Pediatrics* 1996;97(5):669-75.
24. Righard L, Alade MO. Effect of delivery room routines on success of first breast-feed. *Lancet* 1990;336(8723):1105-7.
25. Victora CG, Tomasi E, Olinto MT, Barros FC. Use of pacifiers and breastfeeding duration. *Lancet* 1993;341(8842):404-6.
26. Philip BL, Merewood A, Miller LW, et.al. The Baby-Friendly Hospital Initiative improves breastfeeding initiation rates in a US hospital setting. Pediatrics 2001; In press.

Acute otitis media (Ear infection)

Summary

Breastfeeding should continue unrestricted throughout episodes of acute otitis media. Breastfeeding protects against developing ear infections.

Definition/cause

The eustachian tube connects the middle ear to the posterior pharynx and serves to equalize the pressure in the middle ear with atmospheric pressure, to drain middle ear secretions to the posterior pharynx, and to prevent reflux of nasopharyngeal secretions into the middle ear.   When the eustachian tube becomes blocked or malfunctions, fluid accumulates in the middle ear space.   If this fluid becomes infected, acute otitis media can result.

Ear infections have a peak incidence in the first two years of life, particularly between six and 12 months.[1]   By their first birthday, two out of three children will have suffered at least one ear infection.[2] Risk factors for developing ear infections in the first two years of life include formula-feeding,[3-12] daycare attendance,[3] male sex,[1] low socioeconomic status,[1] smoking,[13] and pacifier use.[14]   Ear infections are also more common in certain population groups like Alaskan and Canadian Inuit and Native American children,[2] and in children with Down syndrome, or with a craniofacial defect such as cleft palate.[15]

Signs and symptoms

An infant with an ear infection may be fussy, febrile, exhibit poor appetite, and may recently have suffered from a cold.   Other symptoms include ear pain, loose stools, episodes of prolonged crying and disturbed sleep.   Sometimes infants pull at their ears or shake their heads due to discomfort, and may pull off the breast while nursing.

Treatment

One ten year review examined the isolates of effusions from 2807 children with acute otitis media.   Sixteen percent has no growth, 35% of cases were caused by *Streptococcus pneumoniae*, 23% by *Haemophilus influenzae,* 14% by *Moraxella catarrhalis*, 3% by group A *streptococcus*, 1% by *Staphylococcus aureus*, and the remainder by other bacteria.[16]

The most common viral causes of otitis media are first, respiratory syncytial virus, second, rhinovirus and third, influenza virus.[17] Until recently in the United States, a 10 day course of antibiotics has commonly been prescribed as the treatment of choice for an infant with an ear infection.   With increasing organism resistance to antibiotics, many clinicians are leaning towards a shorter course of treatment, or an alternative   approach   of   symptomatic   relief   without   antibiotic treatment.[18] Note that antibiotic therapies may increase the chance of a yeast infection developing in the nursing dyad.

Acute otitis media and breastfeeding

Infants with an ear infection should continue to breastfeed.[19] In addition, breastfeeding protects against developing ear infections.[3-12] In one study, infants who breastfed exclusively for at least four months had half as many episodes of acute otitis media as formula-fed infants in the first year of life.[4]

Food for thought

- In the USA in 1996, approximately 30 million cases of acute otitis media were diagnosed.
- The annual cost of treating US children under five years for acute otitis media is estimated at $5 billion per year.[20]
- Researchers compared infants who received only formula for three months with infants who exclusively breastfed for three months. They found that, in the first year of life, for every 1000 formula-fed infants there were 2033 excess office visits, 212 excess days of hospitalization, and 609 excess prescriptions for otitis media, lower respiratory tract illnesses, and gastrointestinal illness compared to every 1000 breastfed infants. Researchers concluded that each formula-fed infant costs the health care system between $331 and $475 during the first year of life.[21]

References

1. Paradise JL, Rockette HE, Colborn DK, Bernard BS, Smith CG, Kurs-Lasky M, et al. Otitis media in 2253 Pittsburgh-area infants: prevalence and risk factors during the first two years of life. *Pediatrics* 1997;99(3):318-33.
2. Johnson KB, Oski FA. *Oski's Essential Pediatrics.* Philadelphia:Lippincott and Raven;1997:135-137.
3. Duffy LC, Faden H, Wasielewski R, Wolf J, Krystofik D. Exclusive breastfeeding protects against bacterial colonization and day care exposure to otitis media. *Pediatrics* 1997;100(4):E7.
4. Duncan B, Ey J, Holberg CJ, Wright AL, Martinez FD, Taussig LM. Exclusive breast-feeding for at least 4 months protects against otitis media. *Pediatrics* 1993;91(5):867-72.
5. Kero P, Piekkala P. Factors affecting the occurrence of acute otitis media during the first year of life. *Acta Paediatr Scand* 1987;76(4):618-23.

6. Alho OP, Koivu M, Sorri M, Rantakallio P. Risk factors for recurrent acute otitis media and respiratory infection in infancy. *Int J Pediatr Otorhinolaryngol* 1990;19(2):151-61.
7. Aniansson G, Alm B, Andersson B, Hakansson A, Larsson P, Nylen O, et al. A prospective cohort study on breast-feeding and otitis media in Swedish infants. *Pediatr Infect Dis J* 1994;13(3):183-8.
8. Engel J, Anteunis L, Volovics A, Hendriks J, Marres E. Risk factors of otitis media with effusion during infancy. *Int J Pediatr Otorhinolaryngol* 1999;48(3):239-49.
9. Infante-Rivard C, Fernandez A. Otitis media in children: Frequency, risk factors, and research avenues. *Epidemiol Rev* 1993;15:444.
10. Sassen ML, Brand R, Grote JJ. Breast-feeding and acute otitis media. *Am J Otolaryngol* 1994;15(5):351-7.
11. Shaaban KM, Hamadnalla I. The effect of duration of breast feeding on the occurrence of acute otitis media in children under three years. *East Afr Med J* 1993;70(10):632-4.
12. Teele DW, Klein JO, Rosner B. Epidemiology of otitis media during the first seven years of life in children in greater Boston: a prospective, cohort study. *J Infect Dis* 1989;160(1):83-94.
13. Owen MJ, Baldwin CD, Swank PR, Pannu AK, Johnson DL, Howie VM. Relation of infant feeding practices, cigarette smoke exposure, and group child care to the onset and duration of otitis media with effusion in the first two years of life. *J Pediatr* 1993;123(5):702-11.
14. Niemela M, Uhari M, Mottonen M. A pacifier increases the risk of recurrent acute otitis media in children in day care centers. *Pediatrics* 1995;96(5 Pt 1):884-8.
15. Paradise JL, Elster BA, Tan L. Evidence in infants with cleft palate that breast milk protects against otitis media. *Pediatrics* 1994;94(6 Pt 1):853-60.
16. Bluestone CD, Stephenson JS, Martin LM. Ten-year review of otitis media pathogens. *Pediatr Infect Dis J* 1992;11(8 Suppl):S7-11.
17. Ruuskanen O, Arola M, Heikkinen T, Ziegler T. Viruses in acute otitis media: increasing evidence for clinical significance. *Pediatr Infect Dis J* 1991;10(6):425-7.
18. Bauchner H, Philipp B. Reducing inappropriate antibiotic use. *Pediatrics* 1998;102:142-145.
19. Scariati PD, Grummer-Strawn LM, Fein SB. A longitudinal analysis of infant morbidity and the extent of breastfeeding in the United States. *Pediatrics* 1997;99(6):E5.
20. Bondy J, Berman S, Glazner J, Lezotte D. Direct expenditures related to otitis media diagnoses: extrapolations from a pediatric medicaid cohort. *Pediatrics* 2000;105(6):E72.
21. Ball TM, Wright AL. Health care costs of formula-feeding in the first year of life. *Pediatrics* 1999;103(4 Pt 2):870-6.

Adoptive nursing

Summary
The woman who wishes to breastfeed her adopted infant should be encouraged to do so, although she may not be able to create a full milk supply.

Adoptive nursing and breastfeeding
A cultural perspective
It is hardly surprising, in a western culture where many women do not breastfeed their biological children because it is 'too embarrassing',[1] that the concept of breastfeeding an adopted child is often greeted with amazement. In fact, since the time of the ancient Greeks (and presumably since prehistory), nursing the child of another mother has been a socially acceptable event. Sometimes the arrangement was commercial, with professional wet nurses hired for noble European families; other times it was prompted by maternal death, or by catastrophic events where breastfeeding was needed to nourish sick or motherless children.[2]

Today, much of the research on breastfeeding non-biological children originates from non-industrialized nations,[3-5] where breastmilk lowers the risk of infection, and can prove lifesaving for motherless or adopted children, or for infants weaned too early from the breast.[6-12] In western societies, however, women who choose to nurse adopted infants are usually mothers seeking to create the nursing relationship with their non-biological child.[2]

Definitions
Relactation is the process of creating a milk supply in women who have recently given birth, but have not breastfed successfully, or have stopped breastfeeding, and must thus 'relactate' to recreate a milk supply. Induced lactation is the process of creating a milk supply in 'nonpuerpal' women: women who have not recently given birth, and who may or may not have previously been pregnant or nursed other children.

Expectations

Breastfeeding has many benefits for mother and child beyond provision of milk.   In one study of 240 women who breastfed adopted babies, the majority stated that enhancing the maternal-infant relationship was the prime goal.[13] Because the outcome of induced lactation is unpredictable, the adoptive mother should be counseled from the outset to focus first on nurture and second on nourishment. Seen in this light, breastmilk is a bonus, but nursing is still successful if the infant suckles and the dyad enjoys the relationship. If 'success' is to be measured in ounces of milk, the mother may be disappointed.[2,14]

On the other hand, induced lactation can produce milk. Lakhkar found that among 12 mothers who induced lactation for their adopted babies, eight initiated breastfeeding, and four of them produced a sufficient milk supply, while four produced a partial supply.[5]   The mean time to lactation was eight days.[5] Another study claimed that of 27 non-puerperal women who completed a comprehensive lactation induction program, 24 (89%) went on to breastfeed 'successfully', including all 11 women who had never previously lactated.[4] Such outstanding results are not typical of other research. In both studies, women participated in an organized lactation program involving counseling, support, and medication.   However as there were no control groups, it was difficult to assess which interventions worked best.

Practicalities

The mother who has not given birth, either recently or ever, induces lactation by breast stimulation. Although her breasts are not 'primed' by the hormonal changes of pregnancy, milk production can occur simply as a result of nipple stimulation. If the date of the anticipated adoption is known, some women obtain an electric breast pump and begin to pump the breasts on a regular schedule before the child's arrival. Although this is a logical first step, the efficacy of early pumping has not been documented. Factors which do appear to enhance milk production include the age of the infant,[3,15] (infants under eight weeks of age were the most willing nursers in one study)[13], and previous maternal lactation. However, simultaneously nursing an older child who has breastfed since birth does not guarantee the mother will create a full milk supply for the newly adopted infant.[13]

In most lactation programs reported, metoclopramide, which has been shown to raise base prolactin levels and milk supply in lactating women,[16-18] was prescribed. Again, a lack of control subjects means its effect was unproven, but based on its ability to raise prolactin levels in lactating women with low milk supply, it would be expected to improve milk production. The recommended dose in lactating women is 30-45mg per day. (See Low Milk Supply for more information on galactogogues).

Even when the mother is not fully lactating, if the infant will latch on well to the breast, she can give all feeds at breast using a supplemental nursing system (SNS™) (see Breastfeeding aids). Infant formula in the supplementer will guarantee adequate nourishment if her milk supply is insufficient.

Food for thought
- The only undomesticated mammal known to lactate spontaneously is the dwarf mongoose.[2]

Resources
Breastfeeding the Adopted Baby. By Debra Stewart Peterson. Corona Publishing Co., US $12.95.

References
1. Matthews K, Webber K, McKim E, Banoub-Baddour S, Laryea M. Maternal infant-feeding decisions: reasons and influences. *Can J Nurs Res* 1998;30(2):177-98.
2. Lawrence RA, Lawrence RM. *Breastfeeding: A Guide for the Medical Profession.* 5th ed. St. Louis: Mosby;1999:633-652.
3. Rogers IS. Relactation. *Early Hum Dev* 1997;49 Suppl:S75-81.
4. Nemba K. Induced lactation: a study of 37 non-puerperal mothers. *J Trop Pediatr* 1994;40(4):240-2.
5. Lakhkar BB. Breastfeeding in Adopted Babies. *Indian Pediatr* 2000;37(10):1114-1116.
6. Golding J, Emmett PM, Rogers IS. Gastroenteritis, diarrhoea and breast feeding. *Early Hum Dev* 1997;49 Suppl:S83-103.
7. Feachem RG, Koblinsky MA. Interventions for the control of diarrhoeal diseases among young children: promotion of breast-feeding. *Bull World Health Organ* 1984;62(2):271-91.
8. Gracey M. Nutritional effects and management of diarrhoea in infancy. *Acta Paediatr Suppl* 1999;88(430):110-26.

9. Dewey KG, Heinig MJ, Nommsen-Rivers LA. Differences in morbidity between breast-fed and formula-fed infants. *J Pediatr* 1995;126(5 Pt 1):696-702.
10. Beaudry M, Dufour R, Marcoux S. Relation between infant feeding and infections during the first six months of life. *J Pediatr* 1995;126(2):191-7.
11. Popkin BM, Adair L, Akin JS, Black R, Briscoe J, Flieger W. Breast-feeding and diarrheal morbidity. *Pediatrics* 1990;86(6):874-82.
12. Brown KH, Black RE, Lopez de Romana G, Creed de Kanashiro H. Infant-feeding practices and their relationship with diarrheal and other diseases in Huascar (Lima), Peru. *Pediatrics* 1989;83(1):31-40.
13. Auerbach KG, Avery JL. Induced lactation. A study of adoptive nursing by 240 women. *Am J Dis Child* 1981;135(4):340-3.
14. Riordan J, Auerbach KG. *Breastfeeding and Human Lactation.* 2nd ed. Sudbury:Jones and Bartlett;1999:555-57.
15. Auerbach KG, Avery JL. Relactation: a study of 366 cases. *Pediatrics* 1980;65(2):236-42.
16. Kauppila A, Kivinen S, Ylikorkala O. A dose response relation between improved lactation and metoclopramide. *Lancet* 1981;1(8231):1175-7.
17. Gupta AP, Gupta PK. Metoclopramide as a lactagogue. *Clin Pediatr (Phila)* 1985;24(5):269-72.
18. Ehrenkranz RA, Ackerman BA. Metoclopramide effect on faltering milk production by mothers of premature infants. *Pediatrics* 1986;78(4):614-20.

Ankyloglossia (Tongue-tie)

Summary
Infants with ankyloglossia can breastfeed but, depending on the severity of the tongue-tie, the mother infant dyad may have difficulty achieving a successful, pain-free latch.

Definition/cause
Ankyloglossia occurs when the infant has a short lingual frenulum, which 'ties' the underside of the tongue tightly to the lower part of the mouth. One study of 1041 newborns found a 4.8% incidence of ankyloglossia, with the condition affecting 2.6 times as many males as females; however 64% of cases were classified as 'mild' and 36% as moderate. No infant was recorded as having 'severe' tongue-tie.[1]

Signs and symptoms

An infant with severe ankyloglossia cannot extend the tongue beyond the gum line, and the tongue appears 'heart shaped' when the baby opens the mouth or cries, because the tight frenulum pulls the tip downwards in the center. Unresolved sore nipples or an infant who is failing to gain weight are possible symptoms of ankyloglossia.

Treatment

Tongue-tie may resolve without intervention as the infant grows and the frenulum becomes more elastic. A frenotomy is a minor surgical procedure during which the frenulum is cut, releasing the tongue. After this simple office procedure, the infant can immediately return to breastfeeding.

Ankyloglossia and breastfeeding

An infant with ankyloglossia has difficulty drawing the nipple well into the mouth, which can lead to a poor latch, sore nipples, and insufficient milk transfer.

While several studies link ankyloglossia with breastfeeding difficulties[1-3], the subject remains controversial: there are case reports of successful and unsuccessful surgical outcomes and many babies with short frenulums breastfeed without significant problems. In Messner's study, 25% of mothers whose infants had ankyloglossia experienced breastfeeding problems compared with 3% of mothers in a control group. In the same study, 83% of babies with ankyloglossia breastfed successfully for two months compared to 92% of unaffected babies.[1]

Resources

Tongue-Tie: Impact on Breastfeeding, by Dr. Evelyn Jain, is an 18 minute video about tongue-tie for the physician and the lactation consultant, demonstrating frenotomy technique. It is available from:
Lakeview Breastfeeding Clinic
6628 Crowchild Trail S.W.
Calgary, Alberta, Canada
T3E 5R8
Fax: 403/249-0156
www.cal.shaw.wave.ca/~ejain/index.html

References

1. Messner AH, Lalakea ML, Aby J, Macmahon J, Bair E. Ankyloglossia: incidence and associated feeding difficulties. *Arch Otolaryngol Head Neck Surg* 2000;126(1):36-9.
2. Berg KL. Tongue-tie (ankyloglossia) and breastfeeding: a review. *J Hum Lact* 1990;6(3):109-12.
3. Nicholson WL. Tongue-tie (ankyloglossia) associated with breastfeeding problems. *J Hum Lact* 1991;7(2):82-4.

Atopic dermatitis (Eczema)

Summary

A mother or an infant with atopic dermatitis can breastfeed. If there is a family history of atopic dermatitis, the mother should be strongly encouraged to breastfeed.

Definition/cause

The terms atopic dermatitis, eczema, and dermatitis and are often used interchangeably. Atopic dermatitis is the cutaneous expression of an allergic state. One of many etiologies of eczema, it is a reaction pattern, involving an acute inflammatory eruption of the skin accompanied by itching, redness, papules, vesicles, patches, plaques, serous discharge and crusts.[1] Atopic dermatitis is one of the most common skin disorders seen in infants, children and adults and often begins in early infancy.

Atopic dermatitis has been increasing in frequency since the 1970s. It affects around 10% of the pediatric population; 90% of symptoms occur in children under five years of age. Some 30-50% of children with atopic dermatitis (infantile eczema) will go on to have asthma, allergic rhinitis or hay fever.[1] The cause is unknown, but potential influences include hereditary factors,[2] lack of exclusive breastfeeding,[3] early exposure to solid foods,[4] and other environmental factors. Food sensitivities are seen in 5% of affected children; common offending agents are cow's milk, eggs, wheat, peanuts, and fish.

Clinical criteria suggestive of atopic dermatitis are pruritus and scratching, flares and remissions, lesions typical of eczematous dermatitis, and a family history of atopy, such as asthma, allergic rhinitis, food allergies, or eczema.[5]

Signs and symptoms

Atopic dermatitis occurs in three stages; the rash varies with age. The *infantile* form of atopic dermatitis, which is associated with a pruritic red, papular, oozing and crusting rash, often begins on the cheeks, forehead or scalp at around two to six months of age, and in 50% of cases, will have cleared by age two or three.[1] In *children* who continue to have eczema, or develop the condition between four and 12 years of age, the rash is drier; dry skin patches appear with a predilection for the extensor surfaces of arms and legs, popliteal and antecubital fossas, wrists, and ankles. Seventy five percent of cases improve by the teenage years, but in 25% the symptoms persist into adulthood.

Chronic disease in *adults* leads to thickening and lichenification of the skin, with likely involvement of the periorbital areas, forehead, and neck. Scratching and rubbing in dark-skinned individuals can lead to hyperpigmentation.   Complications include secondary bacterial infections.

Individuals with atopic dermatitis at any age may have other stigmata. These can include perioral pallor, an extra fold of skin below the lower eyelid (termed atopic pleat, Dennie's line, or Morgan's fold), accentuated/increased palmar markings, white dermographism (the skin appears as a white line with blanched surroundings when stroked firmly, unlike normal skin, which appears red), keratosis pilaris ("plucked chicken skin"), and an increased incidence of cutaneous infections.

Treatment

Treatment aims at maintaining skin hydration, for example with moisturizers and by avoidance of harsh soaps, and using therapies such as sedative antihistamines and topical corticosteroids to control itching. Patients should be educated about the chronic nature of the disease and its tendency to flare up. Allergy testing can be performed and allergenic triggers should be avoided.

Atopic dermatitis and breastfeeding

Women with eczema can breastfeed, and those with a family history of the condition should be encouraged to do so.

Several studies have demonstrated a protective effect of breastfeeding on allergenic conditions[6] in general, and on atopic dermatitis in particular.[7-9] One study demonstrated that the protective effect of four months of exclusive breastfeeding on atopic dermatitis persisted until five years of age.[8] Another study, by Lucas, found that by 18 months of age, formula-fed preterm infants with a family history of atopy had a significantly greater risk of developing eczema than premature infants who were fed only breastmilk.[9] As with many chronic conditions, the exclusivity of breastfeeding, combined with avoidance of cow's milk protein and avoidance of early solids,[4] appear to be important factors in the degree of protection conveyed.

Eczema can occur on the nipple, areola and breast, where it may cause discomfort for some breastfeeding women. Obviously, feeding primarily on the unaffected breast for a period is one solution; if necessary, the mother can pump to maintain milk supply until the other side clears enough for her to continue breastfeeding. A case report from the *Journal of Human Lactation* records how one woman with severe eczema weaned one child at four months due to extreme pain and inflammation of the nipples and breasts, but was able to breastfeed a second child for a much longer period after a strong topical steroid cream and a topical antibiotic successfully resolved her inflamed and infected nipples and areola.[10]

Mild corticosteroid ointments may be used on lesions on or near the nipple for brief periods of time to reduce pain and inflammation and the mother can continue to breastfeed. Therapy with topical steroids should be limited to less than 7-10 days at most, or as directed by her clinician.

Food for thought
- "Atopy" comes from the Greek *atopia* meaning "different" or "out of place".[1]
- Eczema has been described as "the itch that rashes".

References
1. Hurwitz S. *Clinical Pediatric Dermatology: A Text of Skin Disorders of Childhood and Adolescence.* Philadelphia:WB Saunders;1981:39-51.
2. Aberg N. Familial occurrence of atopic disease: genetic versus environmental factors. *Clin Exp Allergy* 1993;23(10):829-34.
3. Chandra RK. Five-year follow-up of high-risk infants with family history of allergy who were exclusively breast-fed or fed partial whey hydrolysate, soy, and conventional cow's milk formulas. *J Pediatr Gastroenterol Nutr* 1997;24(4):380-8.

4.   Fergusson DM, Horwood LJ. Early solid food diet and eczema in childhood: a 10-year longitudinal study. *Pediatr Allergy Immunol* 1994;5(6):44-7.
5.   Harrison's *Principles of Internal Medicine.* 14th ed. New York:McGraw-Hill: 298.
6.   Miskelly FG, Burr ML, Vaughan-Williams E, Fehily AM, Butland BK, Merrett TG. Infant feeding and allergy. *Arch Dis Child* 1988;63(4):388-93.
7.   Chandra RK, Puri S, Hamed A. Influence of maternal diet during lactation and use of formula feeds on development of atopic eczema in high risk infants. *BMJ* 1989;299(6693):228-30.
8.   Saarinen UM, Kajosaari M. Breastfeeding as prophylaxis against atopic disease: prospective follow- up study until 17 years old. *Lancet* 1995;346(8982):1065-9.
9.   Lucas A, Brooke OG, Morley R, Cole TJ, Bamford MF. Early diet of preterm infants and development of allergic or atopic disease: randomized prospective study. *BMJ* 1990;300(6728):837-40.
10. Amir L. Eczema of the nipple and breast: a case report. *J Hum Lact* 1993;9(3):173-5.

Augmentation mammoplasty (Breast implants)

Summary
Women with breast implants should be encouraged to breastfeed. The infant should be closely monitored for appropriate weight gain.

Definition/cause
Breast implants come in different sizes, shapes and fillings. *Polyurethane* implants are no longer used due to chronic problems with shrinkage. *Silicone* filled breast implants have been available for 30 years and have been used by over a million women.[1] Many articles have been written about silicone implants, addressing concerns about leakage, autoimmune issues in the mother, and possible pathological responses in the infant. Since 1992, due to these concerns, the Food and Drug Administration has only allowed silicone implants to be used in controlled clinical trials. This decision was described as "one of the most controversial decisions ever made by the agency."[2] Saline-filled implants are now used.

Some 60% of women have breast implants for cosmetic reasons, and 40% of women use them for reconstruction.

Signs and symptoms

Usually a women will self-report if she has had breast implant surgery, and will know which type of implant was used. However, the authors have experience of women who did not self-report. This possibility reinforces the importance of performing a breast exam, ideally during the prenatal period, on any woman planning to breastfeed, and looking for surgical scars, as well as for inverted nipples and other potential complications.

Augmentation mammoplasty and breastfeeding

Four types of incision may be used in augmentation surgery: infrasubmammary (incision under the breast), periareolar (incision around the areola-nipple), transareolar (incision across the areola-nipple) and axillary (under the arm).[3]   The implant may be inserted directly beneath the breast tissue or deeper, beneath the chest muscle, and success of lactation may vary according to type of incision. In contrast to women who undergo breast reduction surgery, women with augmentation surgery are generally successful at breastfeeding. Nonetheless, the possible disruption of normal anatomy by the incision, or abnormal pressure on alveoli due to a compression effect means that the infants of women with implants should be followed closely for appropriate weight gain.

Significant concern has focused on silicone "leaking" into maternal body tissues or breastmilk and affecting the immune system or causing a toxic reaction in the mother or infant.[4] However, no clear relationship of silicone breast implants to connective tissue disease and no association between silicone implants and neurological disorders in the mother have been found.[5] Case reports of issues in children who were breastfed by mothers with silicone implants and suffering from abnormal mobility of the esophagus or rheumatic complaints are not definitive in causative agent.[6,8] In his commentary in *Pediatrics*, Berlin finds no absolute contraindication to breastfeeding by women with silicone breast implants.[1] According to the FDA, intact implants pose no risk, and women who plan to breastfeed do not need to have implants removed, or to have their breastmilk checked for silicone levels.

Silicone levels in breastmilk are difficult to measure because silicone is present in many products like cosmetics and beer.   However, one study showed silicon levels to be much higher in cow's milk and in 26 brands of infant formula than in the breastmilk of mothers with silicone implants.   Silicon levels in the breastmilk and the blood of mothers with and without implants did not differ significantly.[9]

Mean Silicon Level (ng/ml)		
	With implant (n=15)	Without implant (n=34) (p value)
Breastmilk	55.45 ± 35	51.05 ± 31 ns
Whole Blood	79.29 ± 87	103.76 ± 112 ns

(Silicon level of cow's milk: 708.94 ng/ml)[9]
(Silicon level of 26 brands of infant formula: 4,402.5 ng/ml)

References

1.   Berlin CM. Silicone breast implants and breastfeeding (Commentary). *Pediatrics* 1994;94:547-549.
2.   Council on Scientific Affairs, American Medical Association. Silicone gel breast implants. *JAMA* 1993;270:2602-2606.
3.   Kessler DA.. The basis of the FDA's decision on breast implants. *N Engl J Med* 1992;326:1713.
4.   Riordan J, Auerbach KG. *Breastfeeding and Human Lactation.* 2nd ed. Sudbury:Jones and Bartlett; 1999:494-86.
5.   Ferguson JH. Silicone breast implants and neurologic disorders. Report of the Practice Committee of the American Academy of Neurology. *Neurology* 1997;48:1504.
6.   Levine JJ, Ilowite NT. Scleroderma like esophageal disease in children breastfed by mothers with silicone breast implants. *JAMA* 1994;271:213-216.
7.   Levine JJ, et al. Lack of autoantibody expression in children born to mothers with silicone breast implants. *Pediatrics* 1996;97:243-245.
8.   Teuber SS, Gershwin ME. Autoantibodies and clinical rheumatic complaints in two children of women with silicone gel breast implants. *Int Arch Allergy Immunol*1994;103:105-108.
9.   Semple JL, Lugowski SJ, Baines CJ, et al. Breast milk contamination and silicone implant: preliminary results using silicon as a proxy measurement for silicone. *Plast Reconstr Surg* 1998; 102(2):528-33.

Bacterial meningitis

Summary

An infant with bacterial meningitis can continue to receive breastmilk.

Definition/cause

Meningitis is an inflammation of the meninges, the membranous coverings of the brain and spinal cord. The infection can be bacterial, viral, or fungal.

Bacterial meningitis is usually the most dangerous form of meningitis, and a feared childhood illness, causing death in 1-5% of cases, and long term sequelae in 30-50% of survivors. Ninety percent of cases occur in children between one month and five years of age, with a peak between six and 12 months of life.[1]

For infants between two and six weeks of age, the most common bacterial causative agents are Group B *Streptococcus, Escherichia coli*, and *Listeria monocytogenes*. Beyond the neonatal period the most common bacterial causes are *Neisseria meningitidis, Streptococcus pneumoniae*, and *Haemophilus influenzae* type b. Until recently, *Haemophilus influenzae* was the most common cause of bacterial meningitis in children over six weeks of age. However, the HIB vaccine, which is given as a four shot series before two years of age, has significantly lowered the number of cases due to this bacteria in countries where the vaccine is available.

The organisms colonize in the respiratory tract; some individuals remain asymptomatic. The infection is spread by person to person transmission of the infectious respiratory droplets through coughing, sneezing, and poor hygiene. Once in the respiratory tract, the organism enters and infects the blood stream, causing bacteremia, and seeds the meninges. In severe infections, the spinal cord and the brain become encased in pus.

Signs and symptoms

The infection may begin like an apparent upper respiratory infection, or with the abrupt onset of fever, irritability, headache, stiff neck, hyperesthesia, photophobia, confusion, and seizures. Sometimes a rash, poor appetite, and vomiting are present. Infants with meningitis can present as severely lethargic, sometimes arriving at the hospital limp in a parent's arms. Diagnosis is made by obtaining cerebral spinal fluid (CSF) from a lumbar puncture. The CSF may appear cloudy; analysis shows an elevation of white blood cells and protein, and a decrease in glucose. The culture of the fluid will reveal the organism and help with antibiotic sensitivity.

Long term sequelae range from mild cognitive deficits to retardation and deafness.

Treatment

Prompt treatment with appropriate antibiotics and optimal supportive care are critical. Other infants or children who have been exposed to the patient are often treated prophylactically with antibiotics.

For prevention, the *Haemophilus influenzae* type b vaccine, the *Neisseria meningitidis* vaccine, and the newly created *Streptococcus pneumococcal* vaccine are now available.

Meningitis and breastfeeding

Breastfeeding, or provision of breastmilk by use of an electric breast pump if the infant is unable to nurse, should continue for the baby or toddler with meningitis.

Breastfeeding has long been recognized as a powerful protective factor against the development of meningitis.[2-7] One study found an association between a high breastfeeding rate in the population and a reduced incidence of *Haemophilus influenzae* meningitis five to ten years later.[8] Breastmilk's primary protective effect may be its demonstrated ability to defend against *Haemophilus influenzae* type b[3,9,10] and pneumococcal infections.[5]

Food for thought

- Two classic positive signs of meningitis are the *Kernig* sign – when the leg is flexed at 90 degrees at the hip, it cannot be extended more than 135 degrees – and the *Brudzinski* sign – when the patient is lying supine, the thighs and legs flex involuntarily when the neck is flexed.
- The patient may present with petechiae: tiny, pencil-tip sized, purplish spots on the skin, which do not blanche when pressure is applied. Fever and petechiae below the nipple line are usually

signs of serious disease.

References

1. Schuchat A, Robinson K, Wenger JD, Harrison LH, Farley M, Reingold AL, et al. Bacterial meningitis in the United States in 1995. Active Surveillance Team. *N Engl J Med* 1997;337(14):970-6.
2. Cochi SL, Fleming DW, Hightower AW, Limpakarnjanarat K, Facklam RR, Smith JD, et al. Primary invasive Haemophilus influenzae type b disease: a population- based assessment of risk factors. *J Pediatr* 1986;108(6):887-96.
3. Takala AK, Eskola J, Palmgren J, Ronnberg PR, Kela E, Rekola P, et al. Risk factors of invasive Haemophilus influenzae type b disease among children in Finland. *J Pediatr* 1989;115(5 Pt 1):694-701.
4. Istre GR, Conner JS, Broome CV, Hightower A, Hopkins RS. Risk factors for primary invasive Haemophilus influenzae disease: increased risk from day care attendance and school-aged household members. *J Pediatr* 1985;106(2):190-5.
5. Hanson LA, Hahn-Zoric M, Berndes M, Ashraf R, Herias V, Jalil F, et al. Breast feeding: overview and breast milk immunology. *Acta Paediatr Jpn* 1994;36(5):557-61.
6. Hylander MA, Strobino DM, Dhanireddy R. Human milk feedings and infection among very low birth weight infants. *Pediatrics* 1998;102(3):E38.
7. Lewis BR, Gupta JM. Present prognosis in neonatal meningitis. *Med J Aust* 1977;1(19):695-7.
8. Silfverdal SA, Bodin L, Olcen P. Protective effect of breastfeeding: an ecologic study of Haemophilus influenzae meningitis and breastfeeding in a Swedish population. *Int J Epidemiol* 1999;28(1):152-6.
9. Arnold C, Makintube S, Istre GR. Day care attendance and other risk factors for invasive Haemophilus influenzae type b disease. *Am J Epidemiol* 1993;138(5):333-40.
10. Golding J, Emmett PM, Rogers IS. Does breast feeding protect against non-gastric infections? *Early Hum Dev* 1997;49 Suppl:S105-20.

Biting and teething

Summary

Given a vigilant mother, breastfeeding can continue in spite of biting episodes.

Definition/cause

Biting during breastfeeding is often, though not always, linked with teething. Due to teething pain, the infant chews down on the breast to exert pressure on an edematous gum.

Signs and symptoms

Signs of teething pain can include drooling, swollen gums, erupting teeth, eruption cysts, crankiness, and occasionally mild fever.

Treatment

Teething pain can be mitigated by giving the infant something hard or cold to chew on prior to a feed, by rubbing the gum with a finger, or by systemic pain relievers as recommended by a clinician.

Biting and breastfeeding

New teeth in a breastfeeding baby do not go unnoticed by the mother. Often, peers suggest that this is an appropriate time to wean; a bite adds injury to insult and may spell a painful end to an otherwise pleasurable relationship. In fact, biting is usually a temporary, if memorable, breastfeeding crisis. Toddlers with mouths full of teeth rarely bite.

Whatever the reason for biting, it needs to stop. The mother's initial reaction to being bitten, usually a loud cry and the speedy removal of the child from the breast, may effectively dissuade the infant from biting again. Some infants, however, appear scared by this response, and refuse to nurse for a considerable period; biting is one reported trigger for the so-called 'nursing strike' (see Nursing strike). A few infants seem more intrigued than scared, and may bite again in an apparent attempt to test the mother's reaction.

Ending persistent biting means formulating a way to prevent the baby from repeating this fascinating new trick. Concluding the feed immediately when infant bites, placing the infant well away from the mother, and saying a firm 'no'– is one way of communicating to the infant that this behavior is not acceptable. Pulling the biting baby in close and pressing the nose tightly against the mother's chest to block the airway is widely suggested as a solution to biting. At the critical moment, it is hard to remember to pull in not push off. Gently pinching the child's nose may be a more realistic way of achieving the same effect.

A once-bitten mother quickly learns to anticipate and prevent a bite. Biting often occurs towards the end of a feed; a baby who is busy nursing, with the tongue milking the breast between the teeth and the nipple, is physically incapable of biting. Many mothers report a certain 'look' in the baby's eye, a brief pause, or a clenching of the jaw prior to a bite. Rapid removal of the infant at this point, with the finger slipped into the infant's mouth, can prevent the bite.

Some bites occur accidentally as the infant is falling asleep. As the nipple begins to slide out of the mouth, the baby senses this and bites to retrieve it. Removing the nipple before the infant sleeps will prevent this type of bite.

Food for thought
- Some babies are born with teeth. 'Natal teeth' are present at birth; 'neonatal teeth' erupt within 30 days of birth. If the teeth are loose due to incomplete formation, they are removed to prevent the danger of aspiration.
- In around 400 BC, Hippocrates taught that primary teeth were nourished by the mother's milk: the term 'milk teeth' is alleged to originate from this belief.[1]

References
1.   Schuman A. The truth about teething. *Contemporary Pediatrics* 1992;Oct:57-80.

Breast abscess

Summary
Breastfeeding can continue unrestricted on the unaffected breast. Breastfeeding on the affected breast may require a brief interruption.

Definition/cause
A breast abscess occurs when pus collects in a localized area of the breast and is unable to drain. It is usually the consequence of untreated or unresolved mastitis, and the most common organisms causing mastitis are staphylococcus aureus and streptococcus. Abscesses are rare, but in one study, they developed in 11% of women with untreated

infectious mastitis.[1]

Signs and symptoms

A breast abscess can cause redness, warmth, swelling and severe pain in the breast. Systemic signs include fever and general malaise. Ultrasound is often used to diagnose an abscess.

Treatment

A small abscess can be drained by fine needle aspiration: inserting a needle into the abscess and drawing out the infected fluid. A larger abscess requires a surgical incision through which the abscess drains to the outside. Antibiotic therapy, rest, warm soaks and pain medication are usually also recommended. The correct antibiotic is determined by culturing the fluid drained from the abscess. Because the majority of these infections are of staphylococcal origin, anti-staphylococcal antibiotics are usually recommended.

Abscesses and breastfeeding

Breastfeeding can continue unrestricted on the unaffected breast. Some debate exists as to how long breastfeeding should be interrupted on the affected breast. If the abscess requires surgery, breastfeeding may resume after the abscess has been drained and antibiotics have been initiated, as long as the mother can tolerate the infant nursing on the affected side, and the baby can nurse without disturbing the surgical site.[2] (Milk may leak from the site, but this is not of concern). The infant should be monitored for any signs of infection during the maternal illness.

If the mother finds breastfeeding on the affected breast too painful, or if the drain is too close to the nipple for the infant to be able to nurse, temporary weaning from one breast may be necessary. In such a case the mother should still express milk regularly from the affected site, either by hand or with a pump, in order to prevent severe engorgement and mastitis. In order to maintain a milk supply, and to prevent engorgement, the mother would be well advised to pump the breast from which she is not breastfeeding with a high quality electric breast pump (see Breastfeeding aids) for approximately ten minutes for each missed feed. Clearly the amount of pumping will depend on the age of the infant and the amount of breastmilk the mother is producing: the mother of a newborn will need to pump the affected breast more frequently than the mother of a nursing toddler.

Food for thought

- An abscess, unlike other sore spots or swellings on the breast, is a mass that feels 'boggy' or 'putty-like' when palpated.

References

1. Thomsen AC, Hansen KB, Moller BR. Leukocyte counts and microbiologic cultivation in the diagnosis of puerperal mastitis. *Am J Obstet Gynecol* 1983;146(8):938-41.
2. American Academy of Pediatrics. In Pickering LK, ed. *2000 Red Book: Report of the Committee on Infectious Diseases.* 25th ed. Elk Grove Village, IL: American Academy of Pediatrics; 2000:99.

Breastfeeding aids

Summary

This section addresses aids to breastfeeding which are directly relevant to, or specifically referred to, within the text of this book. Many other breastfeeding aids also exist.

Breast pumps

Swedish scientist Einar Egnell pioneered the electric breast pump in the 1950s, basing his early designs on cattle milking pumps. Today, breast pumps come in a vast array of models, sizes, and capabilities. The most effective pumps are the large electric models, which have adjustable speed and suction levels, pump both breasts simultaneously and, like the infant, 'suck' then pause, in an automatic cycle. The vast majority of pumps at the lower end of the market do not generate an effective enough combination of negative pressure and 'sucking cycles' per minute to maintain a milk supply for a woman who is spending significant amounts of time away from her baby (for example, the mother of an infant in the Neonatal Intensive Care Unit). Types of pumps which fall into this 'occasional use only' category include most hand pumps; small, battery-operated pumps which pump only one breast at a time, and small electric pumps which pump only one breast at a time. Despite the fact that many of the smaller pumps can be expensive, there is tremendous variation from one model to the next in terms of efficiency, comfort level, ease with which the product can be cleaned, and durability. Currently in the United States no legislation exists to set minimum standards for quality among breast pump manufacturers. The Breast Pump Safety Act, (H.R. 3372) recently introduced to the US Congress by congresswoman Carolyn B Maloney, would require the FDA to develop minimum quality standards for breast pumps to ensure that products on the market are safe and effective.

Before a mother invests in a breast pump, and before the clinician recommends a specific type of breast pump, the mother's needs should be carefully assessed. A high quality pump should mimic the infant's sucking capacity, which can reach a maximum negative pressure of approximately 220 mm Hg.[1] At the same time, it should mimic the infant's sucking frequency and generate approximately 50 'suck and pause' cycles per minute. Some small pumps, such as the infamous (and painful) 'bicycle horn' hand pump, with a plastic flange and a rubber suction bulb, can reach extremely high levels of negative pressure. However, small pumps which generate high levels of negative pressure are ineffective over the long term, because they do not produce enough cycles per minute to adequately stimulate the breast.

Only a few small studies have examined the efficacy of different pumps,[2] and they are of limited use because new pumps appear frequently on the market. The research that exists demonstrates, somewhat predictably, that bilateral pumping takes less time than pumping each breast individually,[3] and that large, efficient double electric breast pumps, with adequate pressure and cycles per minute, express a greater volume of milk than less powerful, slower pumps.[4] One study suggests that the fat content of milk collected is higher when an electric pump is used as opposed to a hand pump;[5] another report suggests that bilateral pumping raises prolactin levels.[6] Zinaman and colleagues compared various types of pumps to each other and to natural suckling, in order to evaluate blood prolactin and oxytocin levels 10 minutes after pumping or nursing an infant. They found that prolactin levels were highest following the use of an electric pulsatile pump; these responses compared favorably with those of natural infant suckling. Less effective pumps were less successful in elevating prolactin levels. Maternal blood oxytocin levels did not differ when different pumps were compared with each other or with breastfeeding.[2]

Almost all US hospitals use breast pumps made either by Hollister (formerly Ameda Egnell), and Medela; both brands are reliable and comparable in terms of quality. The top of the line, so-called 'hospital grade' breast pumps are the *SMB* (Hollister) and the *Classic* (Medela), both of which retail for approximately US $1500. According to the manufacturers, the *SMB* generates a maximum negative pressure of 230 mm Hg; the *Classic* generates a maximum negative pressure of 240 mm Hg. Sucking cycles are in the 50 per minute range. Many hospitals rely on the lighter, more portable models made by the same two companies: Hollister's *Elite* (maximum negative pressure 250 mm Hg) or Medela's *Lactina* (maximum negative pressure 240 mm Hg); again sucking cycles are in the 50 per minute range. The *Elite* and the *Lactina* are the pumps most commonly rented by mothers of infants in the Neonatal Intensive Care Unit, or by women returning to work. These high grade pumps are expensive, so most women choose to rent, and if the infant is hospitalized, many insurance companies will pay for electric breast pump rental. Rental fees vary from US $75 per month to US $30 per month depending on the length of the rental (a prepaid six month rental may work out at around US $30 per month but a one month rental may cost around US $75). The mother must also purchase the milk collection kit, a separate item consisting of collection bottles, tubing, and breast flanges, for around US $50. Where lack of insurance is a problem, hospitals bear some responsibility for helping NICU mothers to obtain these pumps.[7]

The next tier of pumps, again made by the same companies, are the relatively new 'personal use pumps', which have begun to replace rental pumps in many situations. Medela's *Pump in Style* (maximum negative pressure 220 mm Hg; up to 63 cycles per minute) retails for around US $275, and Hollister's *Purely Yours* (maximum negative pressure 215 mm Hg; up to 60 cycles per minute) retails for around US $225. Most lactation consultants cite clinical experience and opt for the more expensive models when working with women who are separated from their infants for long periods of time, such as mothers of infants in the Neonatal Intensive Care Unit. Despite this, no research exists to demonstrate that the *Classic, SMB, Lactina* or *Elite* are any more effective in establishing a milk supply than the *Pump in Style* or the *Purely Yours.* Apart from the minimal difference in pressure levels, the main distinction appears to lie in the durability of the motor and the length of the manufacturer's warranty. In many cases, especially among mothers returning to work, the personal use pumps will be adequate for creating and maintaining a milk supply.

Despite the lack of studies, it can be stated with some certainty that, unless the mother plans to spend only minimal amounts of time away from her infant, most other pumps currently on the US market are not efficient enough to maintain a milk supply over time.

Breast Pump manufacturers:

Hollister Inc.
2000 Hollister Dr.
Libertyville, IL 60048
Tel. 800/323-4060

Medela Inc.
P.O. Box 660
McHenry, IL 60051
Tel: 888/633-3528
www.medela.com

The Supplemental Nursing System™ (SNS)

Made by Medela, this device is useful for supplementing feedings at breast. It consists of a rectangular plastic bottle, which hangs by an adjustable cord around the mother's neck, and a fine, flexible tube (in three interchangeable sizes) which extends from the bottle lid and can be taped to the breast and anchored into position. The plastic tube should be placed to hang down very slightly over the nipple, so that when the baby latches onto the breast, the thin tube is also taken into the mouth. As the baby sucks, supplement from the bottle will flow into the mouth along with any breastmilk that is produced. The speed of flow can be regulated by raising or lowering the bottle. The SNS™ retails for around US $45. Less expensive, less durable 'starter' models are available from Medela for around US $15.

The SNS™ is useful for adoptive mothers, for mothers who want to provide any necessary supplements at the breast, and occasionally for infants with a poor latch, although some degree of latch is necessary for the SNS™ to work effectively.

Hospital-made supplementer

In the hospital setting, a supplemental feeder can easily be made by screwing a fine flexible infant feeding tube into the narrow end of a syringe. The syringe can be taped to the mother's clothing.

Feeding cups

Special cups are sold for cup feeding small babies; however a medicine cup or any small plastic cup with a smooth lip is perfectly adequate.

The Evert-It™ nipple enhancer

The Evert-it is designed to help women evert inverted nipples in order to assist with the baby's latch. The plastic tube has a soft silicon flange which fits over the areola, and a plunger, which, when pulled out, causes the nipple to protrude, making it easier for the baby to latch on. The device costs around US $20. Research suggests that physical manipulation of inverted nipples prenatally is not effective;[8,9] the Evert-It should be used after the baby is born if the infant is having difficulty latching on.

Maternal Concepts™, P.O. Box 39, Spring Valley, WI 54767
Tel. 715/778-4723 • 800-310-5817
www.snj.com/maternal/evert.htm

The Niplette™

The Niplette™, invented by a British plastic surgeon, consists of a transparent nipple mold with a sealing flange, attached to a valve and a syringe port. When suction is applied to the inverted nipple, the inverted nipple is drawn out.
Avent America: 800/542-8368
http://www.aventamerica.com

Hospital-made nipple evertors

Many lactation consultants use an inverted syringe, with the needle end cut off and the plunger inserted into the 'wrong' end, to evert the nipple. The smooth (non cut off) surface is placed against the mother's breast, and the plunger then pulled gently outwards to evert the nipple.

Breast shells

These are dome-shaped cups which fit over the breast and under the bra; the flat plastic disk across the base of the dome has a hole at the center for the nipple. Theoretically, as the nipple sits inside the hole, pressure from the disk on the base of the nipple causes it to evert. In fact, controlled trials have found that breast shells, when worn prenatally, were not effective in enhancing breastfeeding success.[8,9]

Haberman Feeder™
This specialty feeder is particularly useful for infants with cleft lip or palate, or with other sucking related problems. Milk flow is controlled by the person feeding the infant, and is released from the bottle-like container into a large soft nipple which requires pressure from the infant, but minimal suction. The Haberman Feeder™ is made by Medela and costs approximately US $20.

Hazelbaker Fingerfeeder™
This device consists of a small, pliable plastic bottle, which can be held in one hand, and a thin plastic tube which extends from the bottle cap and can be taped to the finger for fingerfeeding. The Hazelbaker Fingerfeeder™ is available from Medela and costs approximately US $30.

Hospital-made finger feeders
A finger-feeder can be made in the hospital by attaching a feeding tube to a syringe filled with pumped milk or formula, and taping the feeding tube to a clean finger. The finger should then be gently inserted into the infant's mouth, pad side up, and the infant allowed to finger feed by sucking on the finger and drawing fluid from the tube into the mouth.

References
1. Riordan J, Auerbach KG. *Breastfeeding and Human Lactation.* 2nd ed. Sudbury: Jones and Bartlett; 1999:400:393-448.
2. Zinaman MJ, Hughes V, Queenan JT, et al. Acute prolactin and oxytocin responses and milk yield to infant suckling and artificial methods of expression in lactating women. *Pediatrics* 1992;89(3):437-40.
3. Groh-Wargo S, Toth A, Mahoney K, Simonian S, Wasser T, Rose S. The utility of a bilateral breast pumping system for mothers of premature infants. *Neonatal Netw* 1995;14(8):31-6.
4. Green D, Moye L, Schreiner RL, Lemons JA. The relative efficacy of four methods of human milk expression. *Early Hum Dev* 1982;6(2):153-9.
5. Boutte CA, Garza C, Fraley JK, Stuff JE, Smith EO. Comparison of

hand- and electric-operated breast pumps.   *Hum Nutr Appl Nutr* 1985;39(6):426-30.

6. Milk yield and prolactin rise with simultaneous breast pumping. Ambulatory Pediatric Association Meeting; 1985 May 7-10; Washington DC.

7. Philipp BL, Brown E, Merewood A. Pumps for Peanuts: Leveling the Field in the NICU. *Jnl of Perinatology* 2000;4:249-250.

8. Alexander JM, Grant AM, Campbell MJ. Randomized controlled trial of breast shells and Hoffman's exercises for inverted and non-protractile nipples. *BMJ* 1992;304(6833):1030-2.

9. Preparing for breast feeding: treatment of inverted and non-protractile nipples in pregnancy. The MAIN Trial Collaborative Group. *Midwifery* 1994;10(4):200-14.

Cancer

Summary
Breastfeeding has a significant protective effect against many maternal and childhood cancers. If maternal cancer is suspected during lactation, breastfeeding can generally continue during the assessment period.   External or localized radiation therapy has only a localized effect on the irradiated tissue, and would not affect breastmilk, thus breastfeeding could continue in such cases. If the mother requires the less common, internally administered radionuclide (systemic) therapies, breastfeeding would usually be contraindicated. Radiation directly to the breast area may affect milk production by causing tissue damage.   However, breastfeeding could continue on the unaffected breast.

Definition/cause
Causes of cancer can be genetic, environmental, or unknown. Cancer manifests as a malignant growth or tumor, which eventually destroys and replaces the healthy, functioning cells around it.   Cancer can occur in most locations in the body, and can spread to other sites through metastasis.

Signs and symptoms
Signs of cancer include growths or lumps, bleeding, fatigue, and

pain. Breast cancer is the most common form of cancer diagnosed during pregnancy and lactation, but its appearance is rare, accounting for only around 2% of all breast cancer,[1,2] and occurring in just 0.03% of pregnancies.[2] Symptoms of breast cancer in the lactating woman tend to be overlooked because of the physiological breast changes associated with pregnancy and lactation,[3,4] and because lumpy breasts are common in breastfeeding women.[5] Because of this, a thorough breast examination should be performed as early as possible during the pregnancy to identify any pre-existing conditions.[2]

Treatment

Treatment varies depending on the type of cancer. It can involve surgery to remove the tumor if the tumor is accessible, as well as radiation therapy and chemotherapy to destroy any cancer cells which might remain in the body.

Breastfeeding can continue during evaluation of a suspicious mass, and weaning is not necessary when a biopsy is performed for breast cancer.[5] Breastfeeding can continue on the unaffected breast, and on the affected breast as long as the surgical site is far enough away from the nipple to remain undisturbed by breastfeeding.

Cancer therapies and breastfeeding

The commonly administered external or localized radiation therapies have only a localized effect on the irradiated tissue and would not affect breastmilk, thus breastfeeding could continue during these types of therapy. Internally administered radionuclide therapies would usually be contraindicated for breastfeeding women because they are systemic. However, these treatments are rarely used for cancer except in specific instances (one such instance is the use of I^{131} for thyroid cancer). Radiation directly to the breast area may affect milk production by causing tissue damage. However, breastfeeding could continue on the unaffected breast

Breastfeeding can continue while undergoing chemotherapy treatment in some instances, if a brief wash-out period following administration of the chemotherapeutic drug is used. Most, but not all, chemotherapy drugs are rapidly eliminated from the body. During this period, the mother should pump and discard her milk to avoid engorgement or reduction in milk supply. The patient should consult with her physician closely concerning the medication, its systemic half-life, possible transfer to the infant, and other factors.

Cancer and breastfeeding
Preventative effects of breastmilk
Breastfeeding has a significant preventative effect against many different cancers in both women and children.

Recently published research suggests that breastfeeding long term can have a dramatic protective effect against the development of breast cancer. A sizeable study in the American Journal of Epidemiology found that women in China who breastfed one child for more than two years approximately halved their rate of breast cancer compared to women who breastfed for fewer than six months. Women who had breastfed several children for a total duration of more than six years had a similarly reduced rate of breast cancer.[6] Among American women, commonly cited research suggests that breastfeeding reduces the rate of breast cancer by 25% in premenopausal women, with a positive correlation between duration of lactation and protective effect.[7] The reason for this protective effect is not known, however factors which have been suggested include reduced exposure to cyclic hormones, because breastfeeding suppresses ovulation, and protective effects gained from physical changes to the breast during lactation.[6] Breastfeeding also protects women against endometrial[8] and ovarian cancers.[9] Some studies have also found a link between breastfeeding and reduced risk of uterine cervix,[10] esophageal,[11] and thyroid cancer.[12]

Children who are breastfed have lower rates of lymphoma,[13] Hodgkins Disease,[14] and leukemia than their formula-fed peers. In one study of 1744 children with acute lymphoblastic leukemia and 456 children with acute myeloid leukemia, ever having breastfed was found to be associated with a 21% reduction in risk of childhood acute leukemias. The longer the children breastfed, the greater the protection.[15] Epidemiological studies around early life risk factors connected with cancer have associated ever being breastfed as an infant with a 20-35% reduction in risk of premenopausal breast cancer as an adult.[16,17] Another study found a decreased overall risk of all childhood cancers combined for children who were breastfed as babies.[18]

Cancer in the infant
Cancer is rare among children of breastfeeding age, and little has

48

been published about breastfeeding an infant or young child with cancer. However, there would appear to be no apparent contraindications, and breastfeeding can only do good in terms of optimal nutrition, comfort, and bonding.

Cancer in the mother

Women who develop cancer while breastfeeding will need great psychological and practical support. Despite the increasing number of effective cancer treatments, the diagnosis is always devastating, and its psychological effect on a woman with young children cannot be underestimated. The few studies that have examined cases of breast cancer during pregnancy or lactation paint a bleak picture, primarily because of late diagnosis,[1] which is blamed for the fact that in 70% to 89% of affected women with operable primary tumors, cancer has spread to the axillary lymph nodes.[2] In one Australian study of 382 women of childbearing age with breast cancer, 2.6% were lactating when breast cancer was diagnosed. These women, as well as women diagnosed during pregnancy, had significantly more advanced disease than non-pregnant patients, and survival was poor: none of the 10 survived more than 12 years. Although in this study the adverse outcome for women lactating at diagnosis of their breast cancer persisted despite allowance for nodal status, tumor size and age, most research suggests that survival rates are equal between lactating and non lactating women when the tumor is confined to the breast.[2,3,19]

Case reports imply that women who have been successfully treated for early stage breast cancer can go on to breastfeed future children.[20,21] Some women have successfully breastfed from the treated breast, though other women produced little or no milk in the treated breast. Failure to lactate was associated with circumareolar surgery in some patients. Breastfeeding from a remaining, unaffected breast was generally successful.[20]

Although the question is often asked, there is no evidence to suggest that milk from a cancerous breast could transmit cancer to a breastfeeding baby.[22] Neither is the risk of developing breast cancer increased by nursing from a mother who later developed breast cancer. Researchers concluded that there was no evidence that a transmissible agent in breastmilk increases breast cancer risk.[23]

Food for thought

- Breast rejection – when the breastfeeding infant suddenly and consistently refuses one breast – has been reported on several occasions in women who were later found to have a tumor in the rejected breast. Researchers speculate that breast rejection is related to biochemical changes in the milk due to the tumor, which change the taste of the milk.[1,3] However, breast refusal or preference of one breast can occur with inverted nipples, pregnancy, nursing strike and other common reasons.
- The Tanka (boat people) of southern China, traditionally nurse only on the right breast. Postmenopausal Tanka women have a significantly higher rate of cancer in the unsuckled left breast.[24]

Resources

American Cancer Society
1599 Clifton Rd NE
Atlanta, GA 30329
Tel. 800/227-2345
Tel. 404/320-3333
www.cancer.org

Candlelighters Childhood Cancer Foundation
7910 Woodmont Ave., Ste. 460
Bethesda, MD 20814
Tel. 800/366-2223
www.candlelighters.org

References

1. Saber A, Dardik H, Ibrahim IM, Wolodiger F. The milk rejection sign: a natural tumor marker. *Am Surg* 1996;62(12):998-9.
2. Hoover HC, Jr. Breast cancer during pregnancy and lactation. *Surg Clin North Am* 1990;70(5):1151-63.
3. Goldsmith HS. Milk-rejection sign of breast cancer. *Am J Surg* 1974;127(3):280-1.
4. Kitchen PR, McLennan R. Breast cancer and pregnancy. *Med J Aust* 1987;147(7):337-9.
5. Lawrence RA, Lawrence RM. *Breastfeeding: A Guide for the Medical Profession.* 5th ed. St. Louis: Mosby; 1999:525-27.
6. Zheng T, Duan L, Liu Y,et.al. Lactation reduces breast cancer risk in Shadong Province, China.   *American Journal of Epdiemiology*

2001;152(12):1129-35.

7. Newcomb PA, Storer BE, Longnecker MP, Mittendorf R, Greenberg ER, Clapp RW, et al. Lactation and a reduced risk of premenopausal breast cancer. *N Engl J Med* 1994;330(2):81-7.

8. Rosenblatt KA, Thomas DB. Prolonged lactation and endometrial cancer. WHO Collaborative Study of Neoplasia and Steroid Contraceptives. *Int J Epidemiol* 1995;24(3):499-503.

9. Rosenblatt KA, Thomas DB. Lactation and the risk of epithelial ovarian cancer. The WHO Collaborative Study of Neoplasia and Steroid Contraceptives. *Int J Epidemiol* 1993;22(2):192-7.

10. Brock KE, Berry G, Brinton LA, Kerr C, MacLennan R, Mock PA, et al. Sexual, reproductive and contraceptive risk factors for carcinoma-in- situ of the uterine cervix in Sydney. *Med J Aust* 1989;150(3):125-30.

11. Cheng KK, Sharp L, McKinney PA, Logan RF, Chilvers CE, Cook-Mozaffari P, et al. A case-control study of oesophageal adenocarcinoma in women: a preventable disease. *Br J Cancer* 2000;83(1):127-32.

12. Mack WJ, Preston-Martin S, Bernstein L, Qian D, Xiang M. Reproductive and hormonal risk factors for thyroid cancer in Los Angeles County females. *Cancer Epidemiol Biomarkers Prev* 1999;8(11):991-7.

13. Davis MK, Savitz DA, Graubard BI. Infant feeding and childhood cancer. *Lancet* 1988;2(8607):365-8.

14. Davis MK. Review of the evidence for an association between infant feeding and childhood cancer. *Int J Cancer Suppl* 1998;11:29-33.

15. Shu XO, Linet MS, Steinbuch M, Wen WQ, Buckley JD, Neglia JP, et al. Breast-feeding and risk of childhood acute leukemia. *J Natl Cancer Inst* 1999;91(20):1765-72.

16. Potischman N, Troisi R. In-utero and early life exposures in relation to risk of breast cancer. *Cancer Causes Control* 1999;10(6):561-73.

17. Weiss HA, Potischman NA, Brinton LA, Brogan D, Coates RJ, Gammon MD, et al. Prenatal and perinatal risk factors for breast cancer in young women. *Epidemiology* 1997;8(2):181-7.

18. Smulevich VB, Solionova LG, Belyakova SV. Parental occupation and other factors and cancer risk in children: I. Study methodology and non-occupational factors. *Int J Cancer* 1999;83(6):712-7.

19. Lethaby AE, O'Neill MA, Mason BH, Holdaway IM, Harvey VJ. Overall survival from breast cancer in women pregnant or lactating at or after diagnosis. Auckland Breast Cancer Study Group. *Int J Cancer* 1996;67(6):751-5.

20. Higgins S, Haffty BG. Pregnancy and lactation after breast-conserving therapy for early stage breast cancer. *Cancer* 1994;73(8):2175-80.

21. Burns PE. Absence of lactation in a previously radiated breast. *Int J Radiat Oncol Biol Phys* 1987;13(10):1603-4.

22. Riordan J, Auerbach KG. *Breastfeeding and Human Lactation*. 2nd ed. Sudbury: Jones and Bartlett, 1999:499-502.

23. Titus-Ernstoff L, Egan KM, Newcomb PA, Baron JA, Stampfer M, Greenberg ER, et al. Exposure to breast milk in infancy and adult breast cancer risk. *J Natl Cancer Inst* 1998;90(12):921-4.
24. Ing R, Petrakis NL, Ho JH. Unilateral breast-feeding and breast cancer. *Lancet* 1977;2(8029):124-7.

Candidiasis (Moniliasis/Yeast infection)

Summary

Breastfeeding can continue unrestricted throughout episodes of maternal and infantile candidiasis.

Definition/cause

Approximately 200 species of Candida have been identified, but the yeast-like fungus *Candida albicans* causes 60-80% of yeast infections.[1] *Candida albicans* exists normally in the microflora of the mouth, gastrointestinal and vaginal tract of healthy individuals, however, an alteration in host defenses, or a change the balance of gut flora allows the organism to become invasive.

Conditions associated with candida infections are age, pregnancy, diabetes mellitus, immune suppression, and antibiotic therapy.[2] Less common associated conditions include acrodermatitis enteropathica, phenylketonuria, and Down syndrome.

A candida infection can occur in many locations, but most commonly becomes a breastfeeding issue when present on the mother's nipples or breasts, or in the infant's mouth. If the mother has a vulvovaginal candida infection, her infant may become infected in utero, during birth, or postnatally.[1]

Signs and symptoms

Candidiasis should always be suspected in cases of chronic nipple pain, or in "late onset" nipple pain, when a mother who has previously been nursing comfortably suddenly presents with sore nipples.

On the breast, yeast can manifest as a red irritated area, possibly with satellite lesions located around one or both nipples, and possibly across the areola and beyond onto the skin of the breast. The area may be sore and itchy; the mother classically describes candida pain as "burning." However, the rash of a candida infection is not always visible: the mother may have pain during or between feedings, without any obvious physical symptoms.   In such cases, an examination of the infant may reveal symptoms of yeast, which assist with diagnosis in the mother.   Deep shooting pains to the axillary area or inside the mother's breast may be caused by a ductal candidal infection.[3]

In the infant, oral candidiasis (thrush) appears as white, cottage cheese-like patches on the tongue, palate, buccal and gingival surfaces; it can be difficult to determine if the white substance is breastmilk or thrush.   Thrush is difficult to scrape off or wipe away, and when removed leaves a red, raw, inflamed area.   By contrast, breastmilk is easily removed and reveals no area of inflammation.   In the diaper area, candida rashes resist traditional diaper rash creams, and are vivid red, with sharply demarcated borders and associated satellite lesions.   The infant may be fussy and irritable especially when urine or feces come into contact with the affected skin.

Candida infections are not always apparent in either mother or infant, and it is not unreasonable to treat unresolved, unexplained, chronic nipple pain with anti-candida therapy despite a lack of outward symptoms.

Treatment

Candida can be passed back and forth between nursing partners; both mother and infant should be treated, even if one partner is asymptomatic.[2,4,5]

Traditionally, for cutaneous candidiasis, nystatin ointment has been used, while nystatin oral suspension is used to treat thrush in the infant. However, an estimated 45% of candida strains are now resistant to nystatin.[3] Other agents are clotrimazole and miconazole, which can be applied topically to the nipple in small amounts up to four times a day after breastfeeding.   Gentian violet is a topical anti-candida agent which is regaining popularity, although its bright purple stain may deter use by some women.   A 0.5-1% aqueous solution can be applied to the nipples and put into the infant's mouth once a day for three to seven days. Higher concentrations, or prolonged exposure, can cause severe mucositis (irritation) in the infant.[3]

Because of yeast's increased resistance to nystatin, fluconazole (Diflucan), the first of a new subclass of synthetic anti-fungal agents, is being used with increasing frequency to treat maternal yeast infections.[3,6] Fluconazole is available in tablet, powder and intravenous form.   A single 150 mg oral dose of fluconazole has been shown to be as effective in treating vaginal yeast infections due to *Candida albicans* as intravaginal treatment with clotrimazole and miconazole for seven nights.[7] It can also be used for systemic candidiasis: for example, ductal candidiasis in the breast, which could be treated with a loading dose of 200-400 mg, followed by 100-200 mg per day for 2-3 weeks.[3] Maternal fluconazole therapy is not believed to cause problems in the breastfeeding infant.[3]

Preventative considerations for the clinician include prescribing the shortest possible course of antibiotics in breastfeeding women, and treating symptomatic candida infections in women prior to delivery.

Candidiasis and breastfeeding

Breastfeeding need not be interrupted during episodes of candidiasis, although the infection is irritating and painful, and can take time to resolve.

Candida albicans grows best in sites that are moist, warm and dark. Thus, the nipples should be kept as dry as possible, and creams, or plastic lined nursing pads, should be avoided. The mother should wear cotton underwear as nylon and polyester retain moisture.

Some women suffer from chronic candida infections without obvious cause. If the infection recurs, the mother may want to sterilize breast pump parts after use, as well as anything that comes in contact with the infant's mouth, such as teething toys, bottle nipples, cups or pacifiers. In chronic infections, treatment of the women's sexual partner should also be considered.

Food for thought

• One study found that infants who routinely used a pacifier carried a higher oral load of candida than infants who did not.[8]

References

1. American Academy of Pediatrics. In:Pickering LK. ed. *2000 Red Book: Report of the Committee on Infectious Diseases*. 25th ed. Elk Grove Village, IL:American Academy of Pediatrics; 2000:198:201.
2. Tanguay KE, McBean MR, Jain E.   Nipple candidiasis among breastfeeding mothers. Case-control study of predisposing factors. *Can Fam Physician* 1994;40:1407-13.
3. Hale TW. *Clinical Therapy in Breastfeeding Patients*. Amarillo: Pharmasoft Publishing; 1999:83-85.

4. Lawrence RA, Lawrence RM. *Breastfeeding: A Guide for the Medical Profession.* 5th ed. St. Louis: Mosby; 1999:610-11.
5. Riordan J, Auerbach KG. *Breastfeeding and Human Lactation.* 2nd ed. Sudbury: Jones and Bartlett; 1999:488-89.
6. Hoover K. Breast pain during lactation that resolved with fluconazole: two case studies. *J Hum Lact* 1999;15(2):98-9.
7. *Physician's Desk Reference.* 54th ed. Montvale:Medical Economics Co.; 2000.
8. Darwazeh AM, al-Bashir A. Oral candida flora in healthy infants. *J Oral Pathol Med* 1995;24(8):361-4.

Celiac disease

Summary

Exclusive breastfeeding appears to delay, and may prevent, the development of celiac disease, and should be strongly encouraged among women with a family history of this condition.

Definition/cause

Individuals with celiac disease cannot tolerate gluten in their diet. Specifically, they cannot tolerate gliadin, a protein fraction of wheat gluten, or equivalent protein fractions in other cereals like rye, barley and oats. Gluten ingestion leads to damage on the luminal (inside) surface of the small intestine (seen as villous atrophy on biopsy), which in turn leads to malabsorption. Although the exact cause of celiac disease is unknown, it appears to run in families. Ireland has the highest known incidence of celiac disease with 1:300 people affected; approximately 1:2000 are affected in the United States. Celiac disease was first identified in 1950, and its prevalence is currently declining in western cultures.[1]

Signs and symptoms

The first signs of celiac disease may present in the infant by 10-18 months of age, or more typically in the young child at two to three years. Early, non-specific symptoms may include poor appetite, abdominal pain, and loose stools, progressing to foul smelling, frothy stools (due to fat malabsorption), poor weight gain or weight loss, a distended abdomen, and deficiencies in fat soluble vitamins.

Treatment

Individuals with celiac disease are advised to follow a gluten free diet. This allows the small intestine to recover, and damage is reversed. Ultimate diagnosis is by biopsy of the small intestine.

Celiac disease and breastfeeding

Parents with celiac disease should be informed that their child has an increased risk of developing the disease, and the mother should be encouraged to breastfeed exclusively for six months whenever possible, with continued breastfeeding as solids are added to the diet at about six months.

Several studies[1-3] have linked the current decline of celiac disease in western cultures to changes in infant feeding practices, especially to increased breastfeeding rates and to delayed introduction of solids. One study found that children who breastfed for three months or more showed a marked delay in the onset of celiac disease compared to formula-fed infants.[4]

Although the specific role of breastmilk in delaying or preventing celiac disease has not been defined, when nursing mothers eat wheat gluten, gliadin is often present in their milk.[5] Researchers have speculated that the nursing infant's exposure to gliadin through breastmilk may allow for the development of the appropriate and protective specific immune response to gliadin in the infant.

Food for thought

- On occasions, short stature can be the sole presenting feature of celiac disease.[6]

Resources

Celiac Disease Foundation
13251 Ventura Blvd., #1
Studio City
Los Angeles, CA 91604
Tel. 818/990-2354
www.celiac.org

American Celiac Society Dietary Support Coalition
59 Cuptal Ave.

West Orange, NJ 07052
Tel. 973/325-8837

References
1. Littlewood JM, Crollick AJ, Richards IDG. Childhood coeliac disease is disappearing. *Lancet* 1980;2:1359.
2. Stevens FM, Egan-Mitchell B, Cryan E et al. Decreasing incidence of coeliac disease. *Arch Dis Child* 1987;62:465-468.
3. Challacombe DN, Mecrow IK, et al. Changing infant feeding practices and declining incidence of coeliac disease in West Somerset. *Archives of Disease in Childhood* 1997; 77:206-209.
4. Greco L, Mayer M, Grinaldi M et al. The Effect of Early Feeding on the Onset of Symptoms in Celiac Disease. *Journal of Pediatric Gastroenterology and Nutrition* 1985;4:52-55.
5. Troncone R, Scarcella A, Donatiello A et al. Passage of gliadin into human breast milk. *Acta Paediatr Scand* 1987; 76:453.
6. Groll A, Preece MA et al. Short Stature as the Primary Manifestation of Coeliac Disease. *Lancet* 1980;2: 1097-1099.

Chlamydia

Summary
A mother with a chlamydial infection should receive antibiotic treatment, and can breastfeed.   An infant with a chlamydial infection should also receive treatment, and can breastfeed.

Definition/cause
Chlamydia trachomatis is an obligate intracellular bacteria which can cause a range of clinical diseases in adults and infants. Adult chlamydial diseases include trachoma, which is transmitted by flies and is a common cause of blindness worldwide, but is rare in developed nations. Chlamydial sexually transmitted diseases (STDs) include lymphogranuloma venerum (LGV), and the genital tract infections urethritis, epididymitis and proctitis in men, and endocervicitis and urethritis in women.

The infant born vaginally to a woman with an untreated chlamydial STD has a 50% chance of acquiring chlamydia. Acquisition has also been reported in infants who have had a cesarean birth with intact membranes.[1] The nasopharynx of the infant is the most common site

57

of infection; the risk of developing conjunctivitis is 25%-50% and the risk of developing pneumonia is 5-20%.[1,2]

Signs and symptoms

Symptoms in adult females can include a mucoid vaginal discharge or dysuria, but many women with a chlamydial STD are asymptomatic. Complications in women include perihepatitis (termed Fitz-Hugh-Curtis syndrome) and salpingitis, which can cause pelvic inflammatory disease (PID) and may result in infertility or ectopic pregnancy.

Diagnostic methods include direct examination of a tissue scraping, cell culture, testing for chlamydial antigens, and testing for antibodies. Commonly, tissue from the urethra in men or the endocervix in women is obtained if an STD is suspected.   Because chlamydia is an obligate intracellular organism, a clinician must obtain epithelial cells for culture and not only discharge.   Improved screening technologies mean urine culturing is becoming more frequent.

Treatment

For an uncomplicated genital tract infection in the non-pregnant woman, the first line of treatment is azithromycin (1 gm given orally in a single dose) or doxycycline (100 mg given orally twice daily for seven days).

Azithromycin has a long half life, and some is transferred into breastmilk.   However, levels are not believed to be clinically significant.[3] Doxycycline is a tetracycline antibiotic with a long half life which could potentially cause side effects such as dental staining, decreased bone growth and altered GI flora in infants exposed for more than a few weeks through breastmilk. However, short term exposure of up to three weeks is not necessarily contraindicated.[3]   Standard prenatal care includes chlamydia screening during pregnancy; this is the best way to avoid disease in the newborn.

The infant born to a mother with an untreated chlamydia infection is at high risk of contracting the disease through vertical transmission. The efficacy of prophylactic therapy in newborns however is unknown,[1] and current guidelines leave the decision on prophylactic treatment to the discretion of the individual clinician.[1]   An infant who develops chlamydial conjunctivitis and pneumonia should be treated with oral erythromycin (50 mg/kg per day in four divided doses) for 14 days.[1] Sexual partners should be treated, and patients should be screened for other STDs like gonorrhea, syphilis, HIV, and hepatitis B. A history should be taken for herpes and venereal warts.

Chlamydia and breastfeeding

To date there are no published reports of the transmission of *Chlamydia trachomatis* in breastmilk. Mothers positive for chlamydia have been found to have specific secretory IgA antibodies to chlamydia in their milk.[4] Maternal therapy for a chlamydial infection should be initiated promptly; an infant born to a mother with an untreated chlamydia infection may be treated prophylactically at the clinician's discretion with oral erythromycin or another macrolide.[1] If the child is not treated, s/he should be watched carefully for any signs of infection. Breastfeeding should begin as usual, and no separation of mother and infant is necessary.

Food for thought

- At birth, infants in many countries are routinely prophylaxed with either 1% silver nitrate eye drops, 0.5% erythromycin ointment or 1% tetracycline ointment to prevent *gonococcal ophthalmia neonatorum*, the eye disease caused by gonorrhea. However, this treatment is ineffective at preventing chlamydia conjunctivitis.[2]
- Chlamydia and gonorrhea infect similar tissues, but gonorrhea is a more severe infection, causing the possibility of disseminated disease in both mother and infant.

References

1. American Academy of Pediatrics. In: Pickering LK. ed. *2000 Red Book: Report of the Committee on Infectious Diseases.* 25th ed. Elk Grove Village, IL: American Academy of Pediatrics; 2000: 208-12, 741.
2. McMillan JA, DeAngelis CD, Feigin RD, Warshaw JB eds. *Oski's Pediatrics:Principles and Practice.* 3rd ed. Philadelphia: Lippincourt Williams and Wilkins;1999:895-898.
3. Hale TW. *Medications and Mothers' Milk.* 9th ed. Amarillo: Pharmasoft Publishing, 2000.
4. Lawrence RA, Lawrence RM. *Breastfeeding: A Guide for the Medical Profession.* 5th ed. St. Louis: Mosby, 1999:568.

Chylothorax

Summary

Dietary adjustments involving reduction of fatty acid intake are standard in the treatment of chylothorax, thus the physician may recommend temporary cessation of breastfeeding. In some instances, breastmilk has been fed successfully to infants with a chylothorax, but little research exists on this topic.

Definition/cause

Chyle is a clear or milky fluid containing chylomicrons (triglyceride containing lipoproteins) and lymphocytes which, with digestion, is taken up by lacteal vessels, the lymphatic vessels of the intestinal system, and carried to the thoracic duct, which drains into the circulatory system.

A chylothorax occurs when the thoracic duct is interrupted in the thorax, causing chyle to accumulate in the pleural space. The condition is rare, but in neonates the thoracic duct is fragile and may occasionally leak due to trauma or stretching. Other causes include complications of thoracic surgery, such as cardiac surgery, a malformation of the thoracic duct, or an unknown, idiopathic cause. A study of 51 cases over 12 years found that in 65% of instances, the problem was caused by direct injury to the thoracic duct; in 27% the cause was thrombosis or venous pressure in the superior vena cava, and in 8% the cause was congenital. Forty-six of the cases were diagnosed after cardiothoracic surgery.[1]

Signs and symptoms

As chyle accumulates in the pleural space, infants may present with shortness of breath or respiratory distress;[2,3] there are also reports of birth asphyxia.[2] Chyle is bacteriostatic, so fever and pleuritic pain are not usually seen.

Treatment

Chylothorax is a rare event and some controversy surrounds its management. Upon diagnosis of severe cases, drainage of the pleural space via a chest tube and mechanical ventilation may be required to resolve the initial symptomatic complications.[2,3] Treatment options for the chylothorax itself consist of either a conservative approach, based primarily on diet adjustment and allowing the duct to heal over time[1,4] or a more interventional approach involving surgery. Surgery may be necessary if a more conservative approach fails. One study found conservative treatment to be effective in 80% of infants and children presenting with chylothorax.[1] However, both approaches have drawbacks. Conservative treatment may not resolve the condition for several weeks, and dietary manipulation is not straightforward. On the other hand, surgical intervention does not necessarily provide a more successful outcome, and generally involves greater risk.

If diagnosed in utero, chylothorax can be treated prenatally with an antenatal shunt.[5,6]

Chylothorax and breastfeeding

Because chylothorax occurs so rarely, the studies reviewing its resolution involve small numbers of infants. Reports involving breastfeeding and chylothorax are rarer still. Controversy over chylothorax and breastfeeding exists because breastfeeding may be interrupted as part of the dietary therapy involved in conservative management of the condition. If breastfeeding is interrupted, it may be for weeks or even months.[6]

Decreasing the intake of long chain fatty acids (which are contained in breastmilk) is generally believed to reduce the volume of chyle produced. The infant may receive a specialized formula high in medium chain triglycerides (MTCs), or may be fed by total parenteral nutrition.[3,7,8] MTCs are offered because they are absorbed directly into the portal circulation.

However, dietary changes are not always as effective as anticipated. One study analyzed the volume and contents of the pleural fluid from a three week old infant with spontaneous chylothorax during parenteral, non-fatty nutrition, and later during administration of an MCT containing formula. The authors were unable to correlate pleural fluid production with the treatment method, and concluded that the use of MCT formula appeared to be "without value in the treatment of spontaneous, neonatal chylothorax."[9] Another retrospective study of 15 children aged between three months and nine years looked at conservative, dietary management, and found that the median duration of chyle leak was 12 days, with a range of four to 64 days. Although the authors recommended conservative and dietary therapy over surgical management, they commented, "In our experience, it is not possible to identify any single dietary manouevre that is superior in reducing chyle flow."[4]

Perhaps more significantly for breastfeeding women, a new, retrospective study of all 19 infants treated for congenital chylothorax at two hospitals over 13 years found that 12 affected infants successfully breastfed or ate regular infant formula, while seven infants were fed MCT rich formula. All infants recovered regardless of the mode of therapy. The study concluded that breastmilk and/or regular infant formula should be offered to infants with a chylothorax before switching to an MCT-rich formula.[6]

Food for thought

- Chylothorax in older children has been linked with child abuse.[10,11]
- Yellow nail syndrome is the term given to a condition marked by slow-growing, yellow nails, lymphedema, and pleural effusion, which results from hypoplastic or dilated lymphatics. Two recent articles describe the birth of infants with a chylothorax to women who suffered from yellow nail syndrome during pregnancy.[12,13]

References

1. Beghetti M, La Scala G, Belli D, Bugmann P, Kalangos A, Le Coultre C. Etiology and management of pediatric chylothorax. *J Pediatr* 2000;136(5):653-8.
2. van Straaten HL, Gerards LJ, Krediet TG. Chylothorax in the neonatal period. *Eur J Pediatr* 1993;152(1):2-5.
3. Ozkan H, Ay N, Ozaksoy D, Ercal D, Erata Y, Durak H, et al. Congenital chylothorax. *Turk J Pediatr* 1996;38(1):113-7.
4. Puntis JW, Roberts KD, Handy D. How should chylothorax be managed? *Arch Dis Child* 1987;62(6):593-6.
5. Mussat P, Dommergues M, Parat S, Mandelbrot L, de Gamarra E, Dumez Y, et al. Congenital chylothorax with hydrops: postnatal care and outcome following antenatal diagnosis. *Acta Paediatr* 1995;84(7):749-55.
6. Al-Tawil K, Ahmed G, Al-Hathal M, Al-Jarallah Y, Campbell N. Congenital chylothorax. *Am J Perinatol* 2000;17(3):121-6.
7. Van Aerde J, Campbell AN, Smyth JA, Lloyd D, Bryan MH. Spontaneous chylothorax in newborns. *Am J Dis Child* 1984;138(10):961-4.
8. Fernandez Alvarez JR, Kalache KD, Grauel EL. Management of spontaneous congenital chylothorax: oral medium-chain triglycerides versus total parenteral nutrition. *Am J Perinatol* 1999;16(8):415-20.
9. Peitersen B, Jacobsen B. Medium chain triglycerides for treatment of spontaneous, neonatal chylothorax. Lipid analysis of the chyle. *Acta Paediatr Scand* 1977;66(1):121-5.

10. Guleserian KJ, Gilchrist BF, Luks FI, Wesselhoeft CW, DeLuca FG. Child abuse as a cause of traumatic chylothorax. *J Pediatr Surg* 1996;31(12):1696-7.
11. Geismar SL, Tilelli JA, Campbell JB, Chiaro JJ. Chylothorax as a manifestation of child abuse. *Pediatr Emerg Care* 1997;13(6):386-9.
12. Slee J, Nelson J, Dickinson J, Kendall P, Halbert A. Yellow nail syndrome presenting as non-immune hydrops: second case report. *Am J Med Genet* 2000;93(1):1-4.
13. Govaert P, Leroy JG, Pauwels R, Vanhaesebrouck P, De Praeter C, Van Kets H, et al. Perinatal manifestations of maternal yellow nail syndrome. *Pediatrics* 1992;89(6 Pt 1):1016-8.

Cleft lip and cleft palate

Summary

The mother of an infant with a cleft lip or palate should be encouraged to provide breastmilk for her child. Breastfeeding success will depend on the severity of the cleft, hospital policies concerning surgery and repair, and support for the mother.

Definition/cause

A cleft lip and/or palate is a birth anomaly which manifests as incomplete fusion of the upper lip and/or palate. Clefts may be associated with other, more complex genetic anomalies. Having a parent or a previous offspring with a cleft means an increased risk for clefts in future children.

Characteristics

A cleft lip is very obvious as a vertical gap in the upper lip under the nose. The space may or may not extend as far as the nostril; there may also be loose flaps of skin, and a protrusion of the upper palate, which can extend out of the mouth. While a cleft lip is obvious, on rare occasions a small cleft of the palate may be missed during a newborn exam, and may surface later as a 'feeding problem' (poor weight gain or milk coming out of the nose could be signs of an undiagnosed cleft palate). Half of affected infants have both a cleft lip and a cleft palate, 25% have a cleft lip only, and 25% have a cleft palate only. The infant may have a unilateral or bilateral cleft lip, a unilateral or bilateral cleft palate, or a combination of both. Parents naturally find these facial abnormalities distressing and may be upset or embarrassed by their infant's appearance.   It is helpful for them to see pictures of successfully repaired clefts.

Treatment

A cleft lip is usually repaired by surgery between the 2nd and 10th week of life. Cleft palates are repaired much later, usually during the second year of life. An obturator - a device which fits over the palate - may be temporarily placed in the mouth before surgical repair of the palate is performed.

Clefts and breastfeeding

Breastmilk protects against ear infections,[1] and infants with clefts are particularly susceptible to chronic otitis media and resultant hearing loss.[2] One study examined 315 infants under two years of age with cleft palates, and found that 32% of infants who received breastmilk were free of effusion in one or more ears at one or more pediatric visits, compared with only 2.7% of formula-fed infants.   This difference emerged independently of feeding method: most mothers of the breastmilk-fed infants used pumps to collect breastmilk, and almost all the infants received their nutrition via an artificial feeder.[2]

Feeding is a challenge for infants with clefts, and will take time and patience, however it is approached. Taking this into consideration, the mother would be well advised to obtain a high quality, double pumping electric breast pump (see Breastfeeding aids) and begin pumping within 12 hours of birth to bring in her milk quickly and establish a good milk supply. If the infant is unable to feed at the breast, the mother will need to pump approximately every three hours for 10 minutes in order to maintain her milk supply. Even if the infant is nursing, she may need the pump to provide supplementary breastmilk, and to maintain her supply when the baby undergoes surgery.

The prime feeding problem for these infants is creating a seal, and here the soft, malleable breast has an advantage over the bottle. Infants that are not feeding at the breast, or need to be supplemented away from the breast, often need to use a device with a large soft nipple, such as the Haberman™ feeder (See Breastfeeding aids), which requires pressure but little or no suction.

Infants with cleft lip alone have the best chance of breastfeeding success. As in all cleft cases, an upright position such as the clutch or football hold is preferable because the mother can press the breast upward into the cleft to create a seal, and gravity will help to prevent milk from running through the cleft into the nasal cavity. In addition, the mother can place her thumb over the top of a cleft lip, sealing the space. From an early stage the mother can learn hand expression and express milk in rhythm with the infant's sucks, maximizing milk flow and intake. In some cases, extra milk can be given whilst nursing, via a supplemental feeding device, such as feeding tube attached to a syringe, or a commercial product like the Hazelbaker Fingerfeeder ™.

However the infant is fed, weight gain should be carefully monitored, because early success may be deceptive. For example, a newborn may appear to breastfed well in the early days before the full milk supply comes in, but may be unable to maintain adequate intake by breastfeeding.

Surgical repair of the cleft lip is another challenge for the breastfeeding dyad, and enlisting the support of a Lactation Consultant to see the parents through the process can help. Numerous studies support the case for early repair of the cleft lip and suggest that breastfeeding immediately after cleft lip surgery is not only possible but should be encouraged.[3-5] Studies reveal that infants who breastfeed immediately after surgery recover well and gain weight more quickly than infants fed by other means.[3,4] Because cleft palates are repaired much later, a device called an obturator, which helps to seal the palate, has been used to improve breastfeeding success.[6]

Resources

Children's Craniofacial Assoc.
PO Box 280297
Dallas, TX 75228
800/535-3643
972/994-9902
www.masterlink.com\children

Craniofacial Foundation of America
C/o Terri Farmer
975 E. Third St.
Chattanooga TN 37403
800/418-3223
423/778-9192
www.erlanger org/cranio

FACES-The National Craniofacial Assoc.
PO Box 11082
Chattanooga TN 37401
800/332-2372
412/266-1632
www.faces-cranio.org

Let's Face It
PO Box 29972
Bellingham, WA 98228
360/676-7325
www.faceit.org/faceit/

National Foundation for Facial Reconstruction
317 E. 34th St., Rm. 901
New York, NY 10016
212/263-6656
www.nffr.org

References

1. Paradise JL, Rockette HE, Colborn DK, Bernard BS, Smith CG, Kurs-Lasky M, et al. Otitis media in 2253 Pittsburgh-area infants: prevalence and risk factors during the first two years of life. *Pediatrics* 1997;99(3):318-33.
2. Paradise JL, Elster BA, Tan L. Evidence in infants with cleft palate that breast milk protects against otitis media. *Pediatrics* 1994;94(6 Pt 1):853-60.
3. Weatherley-White RC, Kuehn DP, Mirrett P, Gilman JI, Weatherley-White CC. Early repair and breast-feeding for infants with cleft lip. *Plast Reconstr Surg* 1987;79(6):879-87.
4. Darzi MA, Chowdri NA, Bhat AN. Breast feeding or spoon feeding after cleft lip repair: a prospective, randomized study. *Br J Plast Surg* 1996;49(1):24-6.
5. Cohen M, Marschall MA, Schafer ME. Immediate unrestricted feeding of infants following cleft lip and palate repair. *J Craniofac Surg* 1992;3(1):30-2.
6. Kogo M, Okada G, Ishii S, Shikata M, Iida S, Matsuya T. Breast feeding for cleft lip and palate patients, using the Hotz-type plate. *Cleft Palate Craniofac J* 1997;34(4):351-3.

Constipation

Summary
Constipation is rare in the breastfed infant. The breastfed infant has a soft stool; the stool of the formula-fed infant is firmer, with a higher solid content and higher levels of minerals and fats, and a higher casein:whey ratio.

Definition/cause
A child with constipation has trouble stooling: stools are passed infrequently, and are hard in consistency. The condition is usually temporary but some children suffer from chronic constipation. Harder stools and a tendency toward constipation are associated with formula feeding.[1] In an analytical study, Quinlan found that stools from formula-fed infants had a higher solids content, and contained markedly higher levels of minerals and lipids, but considerably less carbohydrate, than the stools of breastfed babies. Differences in lipids between formula- and breastfed infants' stools were due almost entirely to fatty acids excreted as soaps in the stools of formula–fed infants.[1]

Constipation in healthy, exclusively breastfed infants is rare. However, inaccurate diagnosis of constipation is common, as older breastfed babies enter periods when they may go for long stretches of time without stooling.

Signs and symptoms
Straining, discomfort, and pain on stooling are symptomatic of constipation. *Lack of stooling in the breastfed infant baby is not a reliable sign that the baby is constipated.*

The newborn who does not stool at all should be evaluated for physical and/or organic problems, which can include abnormal anatomical issues such as imperforate anus, or organic irregularities such as cystic fibrosis and Hirschsprung's disease. *Lack of stooling in the otherwise healthy, exclusively breastfed newborn may indicate a breastfeeding problem.*

The healthy newborn should pass several black, tarry meconium stools in the first 24-48 hours of life, after which the stools should become greenish brown (transitional stool) and eventually bright yellow if the infant is breastfed. The stool of the exclusively breastfed baby is yellow, soft, sometimes 'seedy', and with the curdy consistency of cottage cheese. Early stooling patterns are a useful tool for assessing breastfeeding success. According to the American Academy of Pediatrics, the breastfed infant who is receiving adequate nutrition should pass "three to four stools per day by five to seven days of age."[2] Fewer than three stools per day during the first few weeks of life is a 'red flag' which may indicate insufficient milk intake: the infant with few stools should be evaluated and weighed by a clinician (see Dehydration).

As the infant grows, however, stooling patterns change. Between approximately six to ten weeks of age, many breastfed babies stool infrequently, and several days may pass without a bowel movement; however, when stool is passed, it is soft. Parents understandably worry that the child is constipated, but if the baby is growing, eating well, and content, lack of stooling in this period of development should not be a cause for concern.

Constipation and breastfeeding

Constipation is rare in the breastfed infant. Breastmilk has a laxative effect, and in the early days of life, it helps to move meconium loaded with unconjugated bilirubin out of the body, thus preventing enterohepatic reabsorption of unconjugated bilirubin and potential subsequent problems from hyperbilirubinemia.

Casein is the fraction of milk protein that forms the tough curd. Whey, the fraction of milk protein which remains when casein curds are removed, contains lactoalbumin, lactoferrin, and enzymes. Colostrum contains less casein than mature milk, and the casein:whey fraction varies from species to species. In mature human milk, the casein:whey ratio is 40%:60%; in cow's milk, the casein:whey ratio is 80%:20%.[3] The firm, rubbery consistency of the formula-fed infant's stool is believed to be associated with this difference in the casein:whey ratio.

Food for thought
• In older children, the most common symptom associated with constipation is abdominal pain.

References
1. Quinlan PT, Lockton S, Irwin J, Lucas AL. The relationship between stool hardness and stool composition in breast- and formula-fed infants. *J Pediatr Gastroenterol Nutr* 1995;20(1):81-90.

2. American Academy of Pediatrics: Work Group on Breastfeeding. Breastfeeding and the Use of Human Milk. *Pediatrics* 1997;100(6):1035-1039.
3. Lawrence RA, Lawrence RM. Breastfeeding: A Guide for the Medical Profession. 5th ed. St. Louis:Mosby;1999:118-119.

Crohn's disease (Regional enteritis)

Summary

Breastmilk protects against Crohn's disease, and parents with a family history of Crohn's should be strongly encouraged to breastfeed their child.

Definition/cause

Crohn's disease is an inflammatory bowel disease (IBD) characterized by transmural inflammation of the gastrointestinal tract. In contrast to its IBD cousin, ulcerative colitis, Crohn's can involve any section of the GI tract, from the mouth to the anus, and affects the gut in a segmental and eccentric fashion, with normal mucosa existing between inflamed areas. The small bowel is involved in 90% of cases, especially the distal ileum, which is affected 71% of the time. Crohn's is often difficult to identify, with an average one to two year interval between onset of symptoms and diagnosis.

The cause of Crohn's is believed to be genetic,[1] and a combination of genetic and environmental factors appear to interact to produce the disease.[2] The disorder is most commonly seen in whites and in individuals of Jewish descent. It is equally prevalent in males and females, and peaks in two population groups: young adults, and adults in their 60s.[3] Approximately 3.5 new cases per 100,000 emerge each year.

Lack of breastfeeding is a risk factor for developing Crohn's disease.[4,6] Nicotine use is also related to IBD. Smoking cigarettes appears to be associated with the development of Crohn's disease, and to worsen its course, in contrast to ulcerative colitis, where nicotine use appears protective[7-9] (see Ulcerative colitis).

Signs and symptoms

The most common manifestations are bloody diarrhea, abdominal pain, fever, weight loss, general malaise, and fatigue. Commonly, perianal disease such as skin tag, fissure, abscess, or fistula precedes GI complaints. Extraintestinal signs are many and can include non-deforming arthritis, erythema nodosum, renal stones, gall stones, uveitis, oral aphthous ulcers, anemia of chronic disease, digital clubbing, growth failure, delayed bone maturation, and delayed sexual development.

Diagnosis is made by a combination of clinical history and physical findings, laboratory work and radiographic and endoscopic findings.

Treatment

Because of the complexity of the condition, no single treatment approach has proved effective. The goal of treatment is to minimize symptoms as much as possible; to observe the patient for potential GI complications like stricture, fistula, obstruction, infection, or malignancy; to maximize the nutritional status, and to assist the patient with the social implications of chronic disease. Therapies include careful, possibly long-term use of oral corticosteroids; aminosalicylates for colon disease, and sulfasalazine. For intractable disease, azathioprine and metronidazole may also be tried. For sufferers of ulcerative colitis, surgery can provide a cure; this is not true of Crohn's disease, where surgery is only used when absolutely necessary, to remove as small a segment of the bowel as possible.

Crohn's disease medications and breastfeeding

A thorough review of treatment options and their significance for breastfeeding women is presented in Hale's *Clinical Therapy in Breastfeeding Patients*.[10] According to the American Academy of Pediatrics (AAP), sulfasalazine can be used with caution in breastfeeding women. Bioavailability is low, as are published levels in milk.[10] Prednisone is approved by the AAP for use in breastfeeding women, and its transfer into milk appears to be low, although the infant's growth should be carefully monitored.[10]

Crohn's disease and breastfeeding

Several studies have indicated that infants who breastfeed are less likely to develop Crohn's disease later in life than infants who are formula-fed.[4-6,11] Parents with a family history of Crohn's disease should be strongly encouraged to breastfeed their child.

Food for thought

- In a study by James, a strong association between developing Crohn's disease and the eating of cornflakes for breakfast was found. Eating a breakfast of rice-based cereals or porridge was not associated with developing Crohn's disease.[12]

Resources

CCFA: Crohn's and Colitis Foundation of America
386 Park Ave., S 17th Fl.
New York NY 10016
800/932-2423
212/685-3440
www.ccfa.org

Pediatric Crohn's & Colitis Foundation
PO Box 188
Newton MA 02168
617/489-5854

References

1. Cho J. Update on Inflammatory Bowel Disease Genetics. *Curr Gastroenterol Rep* 2000;2(6):434-439.
2. Karlinger K, Gyorke T, Mako E, Mester A, Tarjan Z. The epidemiology and the pathogenesis of inflammatory bowel disease. *Eur J Radiol* 2000;35(3):154-67.
3. Johnson KB, Oski FA. *Oski's Essential Pediatrics*. Philadelphia: Lippincott and Raven, 1997.
4. Bergstrand O, Hellers G. Breast-feeding during infancy in patients who later develop Crohn's disease. *Scand J Gastroenterol* 1983;18(7):903-6.
5. Koletzko S, Sherman P, Corey M, Griffiths A, Smith C. Role of infant feeding practices in development of Crohn's disease in childhood. *BMJ* 1989;298(6688):1617-8.

6. Rigas A, Rigas B, Glassman M, Yen YY, Lan SJ, Petridou E, et al. Breast-feeding and maternal smoking in the etiology of Crohn's disease and ulcerative colitis in childhood. *Ann Epidemiol* 1993;3(4):387-92.
7. Rubin DT, Hanauer SB. Smoking and inflammatory bowel disease. *Eur J Gastroenterol Hepatol* 2000;12(8):855-62.
8. Kozlova I, Dragomir A, Vanthanouvong V, Roomans GM. Effects of nicotine on intestinal epithelial cells in vivo and in vitro: an X-ray microanalytical study. *J Submicrosc Cytol Pathol* 2000;32(1):97-102.
9. Thomas GA, Rhodes J, Green JT, Richardson C. Role of smoking in inflammatory bowel disease: implications for therapy. *Postgrad Med J* 2000;76(895):273-9.
10. Hale TW. *Clinical Therapy in Breastfeeding Patients.* Amarillo: Pharmasoft Publishing, 1999.
11. Thompson NP, Montgomery SM, Wadsworth ME, Pounder RE, Wakefield AJ. Early determinants of inflammatory bowel disease: use of two national longitudinal birth cohorts. *Eur J Gastroenterol Hepatol* 2000;12(1):25-30.
12. James AH. Breakfast and Crohn's disease. *Br Med J* 1977;1(6066):943-5.

Hand-foot-and-mouth disease (Coxsackievirus)

Summary

Breastfeeding can continue unrestricted throughout episodes of hand-foot-and-mouth disease, but the infant may be reluctant to nurse due to oral pain.

Definition/cause

Hand-foot-and-mouth disease is an enteroviral illness most commonly associated with coxsackievirus A16 and enterovirus 71.[1] Easily transmitted via fecal-oral and respiratory routes, it commonly occurs during the summer, and spreads quickly among children, frequently in 'mini epidemics'.

Signs and symptoms

Children with hand-foot-and-mouth disease exhibit fever, malaise, and poor oral intake, accompanied by a rash (viral exanthem) that identifies this illness: vesicular (blister-like) lesions in the mouth and on the palms, soles, and buttocks. Oral lesions erode, leaving painful ulcerative sores. For several days as this uncomfortable viral illness peaks, the infant may be cranky and have trouble sleeping; s/he may try to nurse for comfort, only to pull away due to oral pain. The infant may refuse to breastfeed, and an older baby or toddler may refuse solids.

Treatment

Treatment is symptomatic. Pain medications such as acetaminophen or ibuprofen can be used while the virus runs its course. Giving these medications 20 minutes before a feed, and numbing the mouth with cold water for a small infant, or offering frozen juices, ice cream, and cold drinks to an older baby can help encourage the child to eat or drink.

Coxsackievirus and breastfeeding

Although breastfeeding can continue throughout this illness, in practice it may be difficult because of the infant's oral pain. Some infants may refuse to breastfeed completely, and the mother may need to pump to maintain her milk supply. Older babies and toddlers may well exist for a few days on a spoonfed diet of ice cream, yogurt, and cold juices or oral rehydration solutions until the illness passes.

Food for thought

- Foot and mouth disease among livestock can prove disastrous to dairy and cattle farmers. It affects cloven-hooved animals and is easily spread over large geographic regions. Infected animals in western nations are slaughtered in an attempt to reduce risk of widespread epidemics.

References

1. American Academy of Pediatrics. In Pickering LK, ed. *2000 Red Book: Report of the Committee on Infectious Diseases.* 25th ed. Elk Grove Village, IL: American Academy of Pediatrics; 2000:236-38

Cystic fibrosis

Summary

Women with cystic fibrosis can breastfeed.   Infants with cystic fibrosis can breastfeed, although due to issues with adequate weight gain, breastfeeding is often supplemented with pancreatic enzymes and hydrolyzed formula.

Definition/cause

Cystic fibrosis (CF) is an autosomal recessive disorder caused by mutations of a gene located on the long arm of chromosome 7. Although many systems are affected, CF patients typically suffer most from chronic pulmonary disease and pancreatic exocrine deficiency, which result from abnormalities in sodium and chloride leading to thickened and abnormal mucous secretions.   CF is a common genetic illness among whites, affecting approximately 1:2500; one in 20-25 are carriers.   Among blacks the incidence is far rarer, at approximately 1:17,000.[1]

Signs and symptoms

Many industrialized nations screen for CF in newborns; if a screen is not performed, CF may go undiagnosed in the infant.   *Meconium ileus*, a condition in which the neonate is unable to pass meconium, is noted in approximately 15% of newborns with CF, and may be the presenting symptom leading to diagnosis of CF by a sweat test.   If the infant passes the newborn period undiagnosed, the young child may present with poor weight gain, bulky, foul-smelling stools, and repetitive pulmonary tract infections, chronic cough, or wheezing. Approximately two thirds of CF cases are diagnosed by 12 months of age, but some 10% go undiagnosed until adolescence or early adulthood.[1]

The abnormal secretions associated with CF affect many organs, but the lungs and the pancreas are usually the prime source of problems.   As children reach the teenage years, they suffer progressively greater shortness of breath, inability to tolerate exercise, and chronic pulmonary infections.   The long term prognosis varies between individuals, but depends primarily on the extent of pulmonary involvement and the effective functioning of the pancreas.   In 90-95%

of cases, mortality results from chronic pulmonary infections, and 85% of patients suffer failure of the exocrine pancreas. In the 1950s, few individuals with CF survived infancy. By 1990, the average life expectancy was approximately 28 years of age, with males generally living longer than females.[1] However, treatments are becoming increasingly effective, and survival rates continue to improve.

Treatment

Therapeutic regimens include antibiotics for chest infections, and proactive chest physiotherapy to assist in the removal of bronchial secretions. Pancreatic enzyme supplements are used to treat pancreatic enzyme defect. Much interest has surrounded the possibility of gene therapy in patients with cystic fibrosis. Theoretically, this is a straightforward solution, as the genetic deficiency is well understood, and successful replacement of the defective gene in even a small percentage of the lung cells would greatly improve prognosis. However, the technique has not been perfected and at present such treatments remain experimental.[2]

Cystic fibrosis and breastfeeding
The mother with cystic fibrosis

Women with cystic fibrosis can breastfeed, although their own health and nutritional status should continue to be carefully monitored. A survey of major U.S. cystic fibrosis centers revealed that for mothers with CF, 11% recommend breast-feeding, 8% do not recommend it, 42% make the recommendation according to the health status of the mother, and 32% make the recommendation according to the personal wishes of the mother.[18] As more women with cystic fibrosis live into the childbearing years, more research is becoming available on pregnancy and breastfeeding among mothers with CF. Data are still minimal, but current research suggests that the breastmilk of women with CF is 'physiologically normal'[3] and not hypernatremic.[4] One study of five women with CF who breastfed their babies found that they produced adequate milk and sustained their infants' nutrition.[5]

The infant with cystic fibrosis

Breastfeeding is highly beneficial for the infant with CF.[6] Infants with CF are extremely vulnerable to respiratory tract infections, and breastmilk lowers the risk of infection in general,[7-9] and the risk of respiratory tract infection in particular.[9-17] Nonetheless, the infant with CF may show classic symptoms, which include eating (or breastfeeding) constantly with insatiable appetite but inadequate weight gain, and breastmilk may need to be supplemented with pancreatic enzyme supplements and/or hydrolyzed formula.[18]

Food for thought

*   Although cystic fibrosis was first identified by western medicine in 1938, European folklore had long recognized the disturbing "kiss of doom." An old adage reads, "Woe to the child which when kissed tastes salty. He is bewitched and soon must die."[2]

Resources

Cystic Fibrosis Foundation
National Office
6931 Arlington Rd.
Bethesda, MD 20814
Tel. 800/344-4823
Tel. 301/951-4422
www.cff.org

References

1.   Johnson   KB,   Oski   FA.   *Oski's Essential Pediatrics.* Philadelphia:Lippincott and Raven;1997:302-308.
2.   Goldeman L, Claude Bennett J, eds. *Cecil Textbook of Medicine.* 21st ed. Philadelphia: W.B. Saunders; 2000:401-405.
3.   Shiffman ML, Seale TW, Flux M, Rennert OR, Swender PT. Breast-milk composition in women with cystic fibrosis: report of two cases and a review of the literature. *Am J Clin Nutr* 1989;49(4):612-7.
4.   Kent NE, Farquharson DF. Cystic fibrosis in pregnancy. *CMAJ* 1993;149(6):809-13.
5.   Michel SH, Mueller DH. Impact of lactation on women with cystic fibrosis and their infants: a review of five cases. *J Am Diet Assoc* 1994;94(2):159-65.
6.   Lawrence RA, Lawrence RM. *Breastfeeding: A Guide for the Medical Profession.* 5th ed. St. Louis: Mosby; 1999:475.
7.   Beaudry M, Dufour R, Marcoux S. Relation between infant feeding and infections during the first six months of life. *J Pediatr* 1995;126(2):191-7.
8.   Dewey KG, Heinig MJ, Nommsen-Rivers LA. Differences in morbidity between breast-fed and formula-fed infants. *J Pediatr* 1995;126(5 Pt 1):696-702.

9.   Hanson LA. Human milk and host defence: immediate and long-term effects. *Acta Paediatr Suppl* 1999;88(430):42-6.
10. Forman MR, Graubard BI, Hoffman HJ, Beren R, Harley EE, Bennett P. The Pima infant feeding study: breastfeeding and respiratory infections during the first year of life. *Int J Epidemiol* 1984;13(4):447-53.
11. Burr ML, Limb ES, Maguire MJ, Amarah L, Eldridge BA, Layzell JC, et al. Infant feeding, wheezing, and allergy: a prospective study. *Arch Dis Child* 1993;68(6):724-8.
12. Ford K, Labbok M. Breast-feeding and child health in the United States. *J Biosoc Sci* 1993;25(2):187-94.
13. Golding J, Emmett PM, Rogers IS. Does breast feeding protect against non-gastric infections? *Early Hum Dev* 1997;49 Suppl:S105-20.
14. Howie PW, Forsyth JS, Ogston SA, Clark A, Florey CD. Protective effect of breast feeding against infection. *BMJ* 1990;300(6716):11-6.
15. Victora CG, Smith PG, Vaughan JP, Nobre LC, Lombardi C, Teixeira AM, et al. Evidence for protection by breast-feeding against infant deaths from infectious diseases in Brazil. *Lancet* 1987;2(8554):319-22.
16. Victora CG, Smith PG, Barros FC, Vaughan JP, Fuchs SC. Risk factors for deaths due to respiratory infections among Brazilian infants. *Int J Epidemiol* 1989;18(4):918-25.
17. Victora CG, Kirkwood BR, Ashworth A, Black RE, Rogers S, Sazawal S, et al. Potential interventions for the prevention of childhood pneumonia in developing countries: improving nutrition. *Am J Clin Nutr* 1999;70(3):309-20.
18. Luder E, Kattan M, Tanzer-Torres G, Bonforte RJ. Current recommendations for breast-feeding in cystic fibrosis centers. *Am J Dis Child* 1990;144(10):1153-6.

Dehydration

Summary

Breastfeeding can continue when the infant is dehydrated, but fluids other than breastmilk, and electrolyte replacement, may be necessary.

Definition/cause

Because the immature kidney of the premature infant, the newborn, or the young child cannot maximally concentrate urine or reserve water, infants and young children are particularly susceptible to volume depletion, and to accompanying rapid dehydration from common conditions involving excessive fluid loss, such as gastroenteritis and vomiting. The three categories of dehydration, based on the serum sodium finding, are isotonic (serum sodium 130-150 mEq/L), hypotonic (serum sodium <130 mEq/L), and hypertonic (serum sodium >150 mEq/L).

In the newborn period particularly, fewer than eight breastfeeds in 24 hours, limiting time at the breast, scheduling feeds, a poor latch, overuse of pacifiers, and the influence of non-supportive hospital routines can jeopardize effective breastfeeding, and over time may lead to dehydration in the exclusively breastfed infant.[1-4]

In less common situations, an underlying maternal condition,[5] or a neurological problem causing poor or dysfunctional infant feeding may result in dehydration.

Signs and symptoms

Weight loss in the newborn infant is normal, as the infant is born with excess body fluid, and an initial weight loss of 7% or less is not an indicator of dehydration. However, a weight loss of over 7%, a lack of urination, and orange/red uric acid crystals in the diaper may indicate dehydration in the newborn. In addition, the dehydrated newborn may have dry mucous membranes, and may be excessively sleepy and difficult to feed.

If the clinician is receiving telephone information from the mother of a young infant, descriptions indicative of dehydration might include fewer than three stools in 24 hours, scant urine output (fewer than six to eight wet diapers per day), sleepiness, difficulty feeding, and the presence of uric acid crystals in the diaper. If such signs are described, the mother should be advised to take the infant to the clinician's office for a weight check.

Birth weight should be regained by no later than two weeks of life. Once the initial weight loss is regained, ideally, the clinician will be able to calculate the severity of dehydration by calculating the percentile of body weight lost over the period of concern: a 3-5% loss indicates mild dehydration; 6-10% indicates moderate dehydration, and >10% indicates severe dehydration. If exact weights are unavailable, the clinician will need to rely on history and clinical findings. Mild dehydration is characterized by thirst and behavioral changes; severe dehydration may result in shock. Other signs of dehydration can include clammy skin, and a change in skin turgor; delayed capillary refill; dryness of lips and buccal mucosa; lack of tearing; sunken eye position; sunken fontanel; irritability; increased pulse rate; low blood pressure, and scant urine output. Often, dehydration goes hand in hand with hyperbilirubinemia.

The parents may be unaware of the problem: in case reports, severe dehydration often comes as a secondary diagnosis,[2] with parents describing a 'good' or 'quiet' baby who rarely cries, takes long naps, and sleeps for long periods at night. The fact that severe dehydration can go unnoticed by parents underscores the need for early clinical follow up and weight checks for all breastfed infants.

Treatment

The primary goal of treatment for severe dehydration is to restore and preserve cardiovascular function, so brain and kidneys are perfused and can provide adaptive mechanisms to help correct the problem. An intravenous bolus of isotonic fluid (such as normal saline or Ringer's lactate) is usually given. Thereafter, rehydration aims to replace fluid and electrolyte deficits, and to maintain fluid therapy.

An infant who is mildly dehydrated may not need to be hospitalized, but will need supplemental fluids – pumped breastmilk, or infant formula – after each breastfeed, until the danger of dehydration is past. Pacifiers should be eliminated because they encourage non-nutritive sucking: any energy spent sucking should be used to gain milk from the breast. At the same time, an infant who is using a pacifier may fail to give feeding cues, such as rooting and finger sucking, to the parents, and may sleep for long periods without eating, all of which will decrease milk intake. The dehydrated infant should be offered as much supplement as s/he will take as often as s/he will take it, and the mother should use a high quality electric breast pump after each feed to increase milk supply. If the parents wish to avoid bottles, supplements can be offered after the feed by cup or syringe. They can also be offered using the Supplemental Nursing System ™ (see Breastfeeding aids). If the infant is able to latch and suck, using the SNS™ is a good option because the infant is still receiving all nourishment at the breast. Usually (where dehydration has been caused by insufficient breastfeeding), as the rehydrated infant gains strength and begins to nurse more effectively, the mother's milk supply rebounds with the additional stimulation. Supplements can slowly be eliminated while weight gain is monitored.

If the mother's milk supply does not rebound with a combination of extra feeding and pumping, maternal factors should be more thoroughly examined (see Low milk supply).

Dehydration and breastfeeding

In industrialized nations, 'scare stories' linking breastfeeding and dehydration in the popular press and in TV soap operas, are common. This is ironic, because in the non-industrialized world, bottle-fed infants die from dehydration far greater numbers, due to the downward spiral of diarrhea, dehydration, and death.[6-10] In industrialized nations, breastfeeding education and careful follow up of at-risk mothers could dramatically reduce, if not eliminate, dehydration among healthy breastfeeding infants.[2,4]

Descriptions of severe cases of dehydration often follow a familiar pattern, with specific 'red flag' indicators such as those reported in *Pediatrics* by Cooper and colleagues in a retrospective case series examining five infants admitted to a Cincinnati children's hospital with severe breastfeeding malnutrition and hypernatremia. All five infants, who were admitted into hospital with weight losses between 14 and 32%, were born to primiparas. Four were born at term and one was born at 36 weeks gestation. None of the presenting complaints concerned dehydration, although three mothers had called their pediatrician's office with breastfeeding concerns. However, none of the infants, whose ages on readmission ranged from five to 14 days, had been seen by a physician since the initial hospital discharge. Only one infant had nursed in the birthing room; in general, breastfeeding sessions were scheduled by the mothers, who reported that most of the time the infants fell asleep at breast. Three women had inverted nipples and reported latch-on difficulties in the hospital. As a result of the dehydration, three infants suffered severe consequences: two developed multiple cerebral infarctions, and one infant underwent a leg amputation.

Situations such as these could be prevented by clinician and parental education, by an early follow up of the breastfed infant, and by implementation of breastfeeding-friendly hospital policies such as those described in the *Ten Steps to Successful Breastfeeding*. Specifically, from the first day postpartum, the mother should breastfeed frequently, with an initial feed within one hour of birth; bottles and pacifiers should be avoided, no time limits should be set on the nursing sessions, and the infant's weight and early output of stool and urine should be closely monitored.   A weight loss above 7% in the first two to three days of life is an early indication that breastfeeding is not going well.[1]

By day two to three postpartum the neonate should be feeding at least eight times in 24 hours, and should be alert and sucking actively for a significant portion of the feed.   The infant should be well latched on to the breast, with a significant amount of tissue in the mouth, and without causing pain or damage to the mother's nipples.   During the mother's hospital stay, an experienced nurse or clinician should perform a thorough assessment of nursing technique.   An incorrect latch may be as obvious as poor positioning, with the infant feeding on the tip of the nipple, or as complex as an infant who is tongue-sucking without any obvious outward signs of poor latch.   Parents should be taught to look for a minimum of three or more yellowish stools in 24 hours once the baby is older than 72 hours, and should be advised to call the clinician's office if stool counts fall and/or the infant does not feed effectively at least eight times in 24 hours.

Food for thought

- Infants born between 35 and 37 weeks gestational age and discharged home directly may be prone to dehydration because of sleepiness and immature suck.   These young infants should be carefully monitored for weight gain, and the mother may need extra breastfeeding support: it can be unrealistic to expect them to go home and breastfeed in the same manner as term neonates.   If the baby is sleepy, the mother should use a high quality breast pump early, in order to boost her supply and have a supply of pumped breastmilk ready in case the infant proves an inefficient feeder.   Supplements (preferably of breastmilk, and preferably given by cup or syringe) may well be necessary even with the most determined mother, because not all infants of 35-37 weeks' gestational age can breastfeed efficiently.   The use of a pacifier should be discouraged: if the child needs to suck, s/he should be sucking on the breast.   As the immature infant approaches 40 weeks gestational age, s/he will gain strength and should be able to nurse more effectively.

References
1.   DeMarzo S, Seacat I, Neifert M. Initial weight loss and return to birth-weight criteria for breast-fed infants: Challenging the "rules of thumb". *Am J Dis Child* 1991;145(402).

2.   Cooper WO, Atherton HD, Kahana M, Kotagal UR. Increased incidence of severe breastfeeding malnutrition and hypernatremia in a metropolitan area. *Pediatrics* 1995;96(5 Pt 1):957-60.
3.   Clarke TA, Markarian M, Griswold W, Mendoza S. Hypernatremic dehydration resulting from inadequate breast-feeding. *Pediatrics* 1979;63(6):931-2.
4.   Rowland TW, Zori RT, Lafleur WR, Reiter EO. Malnutrition and hypernatremic dehydration in breast-fed infants. *JAMA* 1982;247(7):1016-7.
5.   Kaplan JA, Siegler RW, Schmunk GA. Fatal hypernatremic dehydration in exclusively breast-fed newborn infants due to maternal lactation failure. *Am J Forensic Med Pathol* 1998;19(1):19-22.
6.   Banajeh SM, Hussein RF. The impact of breastfeeding on serum electrolytes in infants hospitalized with severe dehydrating diarrhoea in Yemen. *Ann Trop Paediatr* 1999;19(4):371-6.
7.   Victora CG, Smith PG, Vaughan JP, Nobre LC, Lombardi C, Teixeira AM, et al. Evidence for protection by breast-feeding against infant deaths from infectious diseases in Brazil. *Lancet* 1987;2(8554):319-22.
8.   Brown KH, Black RE, Lopez de Romana G, Creed de Kanashiro H. Infant-feeding practices and their relationship with diarrheal and other diseases in Huascar (Lima), Peru. *Pediatrics* 1989;83(1):31-40.
9.   Clemens J, Elyazeed RA, Rao M, Savarino S, Morsy BZ, Kim Y, et al. Early initiation of breastfeeding and the risk of infant diarrhea in rural Egypt. *Pediatrics* 1999;104(1):e3.
10. Dewey KG, Heinig MJ, Nommsen-Rivers LA. Differences in morbidity between breast-fed and formula-fed infants. *J Pediatr* 1995;126(5 Pt 1):696-702.

Diabetes

Summary

A mother or baby with diabetes can breastfeed. If there is a family history of diabetes mellitus, the mother should be supported and encouraged to breastfeed exclusively, and should avoid introduction of formula or other cow's milk products, particularly for the first 12 months postpartum.

Definition/cause

Diabetes is a chronic disease due to an absolute or relative deficiency of insulin and its affect on lipid and carbohydrate metabolism. Diabetes is classified into types 1 and 2; 10% of diabetics suffer from type 1 diabetes and 90% from type 2.[1]

Type 1, or insulin dependent diabetes mellitus (IDDM), most commonly presents in children and adolescents, and appears to have a genetic component. In IDDM, destruction of the pancreatic beta cells, which produce insulin, leads to insulin deficiency. By the time symptoms appear and diagnosis is made, 80-90% of beta cells have been destroyed.[2] IDDM is a chronic disease, associated with serious complications, which can include autoimmune diseases (especially thyroid dysfunction), limited joint mobility, retinopathy, nephropathy, neuropathy and macrovascular complications. Possible triggers for IDDM include short duration of breastfeeding, or lack of exclusive breastfeeding,[3-8] early introduction of cow's milk protein,[5-8] viral infections,[8,9] and environmental toxins.[9] Risk of having a baby with IDDM is also greater among mothers with type 1 diabetes, older mothers, and women who develop preeclampsia during pregnancy.[4]

Type 2 or non-insulin dependent diabetes mellitus (NIDDM) usually presents in adults and is associated with obesity.   In this type of diabetes, insulin is produced but the cells' insulin receptor does not respond to it.   Gestational diabetes manifests as impaired glucose tolerance in approximately 2% of previously healthy women during pregnancy. Onset is usually during the second or third trimester, when pregnancy-associated insulin antagonistic hormones peak. The diabetes usually disappears after the mother gives birth, however, 30-40% of affected women develop NIDDM within five to ten years.   Although gestational diabetes is usually mild in the mother, aggressive treatment including insulin therapy is often used, in order to prevent potentially dangerous complications of hyperglycemia in the fetus.[10]

Signs and symptoms

Classic symptoms of IDDM are weight loss, lethargy, and polyuria, polydipsia and polyphagia due to hyperglycemia. Diabetes mellitus should be considered in an individual who appears ill, has a history of poor oral intake and signs of dehydration, but continues to urinate frequently.

Obesity is common in NIDDM patients, and weight control by appropriate diet and physical activity is important.

A urine dipstick test may reveal glucose and ketones. Classic clinical findings and a random plasma glucose of ≥200 mg/dl are diagnostic. For an asymptomatic individual, diagnosis can be made with repeated elevations of fasting plasma glucose levels or via abnormalities noted on a glucose tolerance test.[9]

Treatment

Treatment consists of education, dietary management, weight loss where required, and insulin administration as indicated. For IDDM sufferers, exogenous insulin repletion is necessary.

High saturated fat intake appears to be associated with insulin resistance, obesity and increased risk of NIDDM, and diets high in carbohydrate seem to protect from glucose intolerance and diabetes, due to their high fiber content.[2]

Medications used for NIDDM include oral antidiabetic agents such as sulfonylureas, which work primarily by stimulating release of insulin from beta cells. Chlorpropamide and tolbutamide have traditionally been used; second generation sulfonylureas glipizide and glyburide are effective in smaller doses. Metformin and pioglitazone may also be given, but are only effective in insulin resistance diabetics, such as some cases of NIDDM.

Diabetes medications and breastfeeding

A thorough review of medication use in breastfeeding women with diabetes can be found in Hale's *Clinical Therapy in Breastfeeding Patients*.[1] Exogenous insulin is not problematic: the insulin molecule is too large to transfer into human milk.[1] Because breastmilk is synthesized from maternal stores, plasma glucose levels in IDDM women are lower than average during lactation, and many women find a reduced need for insulin while breastfeeding.[11]

However, the study of breastfeeding and oral antidiabetic agents used in NIDDM is limited.[1] The sulfonylurea tolbutamide is approved by the American Academy of Pediatrics (AAP) for use in breastfeeding women, but newer sulfonylureas have not been studied. To date there are no reports of hypoglycemia in the infants of diabetics using such medications, but due to the sparsity of information, mothers and infants should be closely monitored.[1] Unfortunately, data is not yet available on the medications used to treat insulin resistant diabetics, such as metformin, or the thiazolindinedione family (such as pioglitazone or rosiglitazone). However, these medications do not lower plasma glucose levels in normal, non-diabetic individuals.

Diabetes and breastfeeding

Diabetic women can breastfeed. Although not all studies have been consistent, a significant amount of research suggests that breastfeeding, and avoidance of the early introduction of cow's milk protein, appear to protect against the development of IDDM. Because children of diabetics run a higher than average chance of developing the disease,[4] exclusive breastfeeding should be strongly encouraged among women with IDDM. However, issues including medications and high risk births may complicate the breastfeeding situation in the early days.

Protective effects

A number of studies show a dose-related protective effect of exclusive breastfeeding against type 1 diabetes.[4-8,12] Typical of such research is a Finnish study of 103 children under seven years of age diagnosed with IDDM, who were matched with controls. The risk of IDDM significantly decreased among children breastfed for at least seven months, or who breastfed exclusively for three to four months. Children who were greater than or equal to four months of age when of supplementary formula was introduced had a lower risk of developing IDDM.[12]

Almost all research to date has examined individuals with IDDM, however, one study, published in *Lancet*, found a similar protective effect of breastfeeding for NIDDM.   That study looked at 720 Pima Indians aged between 10 and 39 years, and found that individuals who had been exclusively breastfed had significantly lower rates of NIDDM than those who were exclusively bottle-fed in all age-groups. The odds ratio for NIDDM in exclusively breastfed individuals, compared with those exclusively bottle-fed, was 0.41 (95% CI 0.18-0.93) adjusted for age, sex, birthdate, parental diabetes, and birthweight. The study concluded, "The increase in prevalence of diabetes in some populations may be due to the concomitant decrease in breastfeeding."[3]

The other side of the exclusive breastfeeding coin is the

implication that early introduction of cow's milk protein, and by definition, the early introduction of cow's milk based infant formulas, increases the risk of developing IDDM.[6-8,12-14]

Practical considerations postpartum

The chance of birth complications increases among diabetic women. One study of 530 infants born to women with diabetes found that 47% of the newborns were admitted to the neonatal intensive care unit (NICU) due to respiratory distress syndrome (RDS), prematurity, hypoglycemia, or congenital anomalies.   Hypoglycemia was documented in 27% of the neonates, and 34% had RDS, while 36% were large for gestational age.   Twenty two percent of infants were born between 34 and 37 weeks of gestation, and 14% were born before 34 weeks' gestation.[15] Diabetic mothers are also more likely than other women to have a cesarean birth.[16] Because of such complications, breastfeeding infants of diabetics tend to receive their first breastfeed later than infants of non diabetic women.[17]

To maximize the chances of exclusive breastfeeding and breastfeeding success, healthy infants of diabetic mothers should be allowed to breastfeed within the first hour of life, and should remain with the mother as much possible during the hospital stay. Research suggests that allowing mother and infant to remain together uninterrupted for at least one hour after birth, and practicing 'rooming in' policies, results in more successful breastfeeding and longer breastfeeding duration.[18,19] Early breastfeeding will help to offset the high risk of hypoglycemia these infants face.

If the birth proves complicated, and the newborn is admitted to the NICU, or is separated from the mother for other medical reasons, the mother should be provided with a hospital grade electric breast pump postpartum, and should begin to pump as soon as possible in order to create and maintain her milk supply. Any milk pumped should be given to the infant. The mother who anticipates a difficult birth may want to ensure prenatally that a pump will be available for her use. She should pump approximately every three hours for ten minutes, until the infant is able to breastfeed directly.

Longer term considerations

For optimal lactation outcome in IDDM women, attention should be paid to adequate maternal calories, blood sugar control, early breast stimulation, and mastitis monitoring.[17]   The diabetic mother should also be watched for candidiasis, because she is at above average risk for this infection.[11]

Food for thought

* Finland has the highest incidence of childhood IDDM in the world.[12]
* Icelandic cows have a lower fraction of A1 and B beta-caseins in their milk than Scandinavian cows.   This may explain the lower incidence of IDDM in Iceland than in Scandinavia.[20]

Resources

American Diabetes Association
National Service Center
1660 Duke St
Alexandria, VA 22314
Tel. 800/342-2383
Tel. 703/549-1500
www.diabetes.org

References

1. Hale TW.   *Clinical   Therapy   in Breastfeeding Patients.* Amarillo:Pharmasoft Publishing, 1999:60-61.
2. Virtanen SM, Aro A. Dietary factors in the aetiology of diabetes. *Ann Med* 1994;26(6):469-78.
3. Pettitt DJ, Forman MR, Hanson RL, Knowler WC, Bennett PH. Breastfeeding and incidence of non-insulin-dependent diabetes mellitus in Pima Indians. *Lancet* 1997;350(9072):166-8.
4. McKinney PA, Parslow R, Gurney KA, Law GR, Bodansky HJ, Williams R. Perinatal and neonatal determinants of childhood type 1 diabetes. A case-control study in Yorkshire, U.K. *Diabetes Care* 1999;22(6):928-32.
5. Mayer EJ, Hamman RF, Gay EC, Lezotte DC, Savitz DA, Klingensmith GJ. Reduced risk of IDDM among breast-fed children. The Colorado IDDM Registry. *Diabetes* 1988;37(12):1625-32.
6. Gimeno SG, de Souza JM. IDDM and milk consumption. A case-control study in Sao Paulo, Brazil. *Diabetes Care* 1997;20(8):1256-60.
7. Perez-Bravo F, Carrasco E, Gutierrez-Lopez MD, Martinez MT, Lopez G, de los Rios MG. Genetic predisposition and environmental factors leading to the development of insulin-dependent diabetes mellitus in Chilean

children. *J Mol Med* 1996;74(2):105-9.
8. Verge CF, Howard NJ, Irwig L, Simpson JM, Mackerras D, Silink M. Environmental factors in childhood IDDM. A population-based, case-control study. *Diabetes Care* 1994;17(12):1381-9.
9. Plotnick L. Insulin-Dependent Diabetes Mellitus. *Pediatrics in Review* 1994;15:137-148.
10. Goldeman L, Claude Bennett J, eds. *Cecil Textbook of Medicine.* 21st ed. Philadelphia: W.B. Saunders; 2000:1263-85.
11. Lawrence RA, Lawrence RM. *Breastfeeding: A Guide for the Medical Profession.* 5th ed. St. Louis: Mosby, 1999:515-21.
12. Virtanen SM, Rasanen L, Aro A, Lindstrom J, Sippola H, Lounamaa R, et al. Infant feeding in Finnish children less than 7 yr of age with newly diagnosed IDDM. Childhood Diabetes in Finland Study Group. *Diabetes Care* 1991;14(5):415-7.
13. Gerstein HC. Cow's milk exposure and type I diabetes mellitus. A critical overview of the clinical literature. *Diabetes Care* 1994;17(1):13-9.
14. Virtanen SM, Rasanen L, Ylonen K, Aro A, Clayton D, Langholz B, et al. Early introduction of dairy products associated with increased risk of IDDM in Finnish children. The Childhood in Diabetes in Finland Study Group. *Diabetes* 1993;42(12):1786-90.
15. Cordero L, Treuer SH, Landon MB, Gabbe SG. Management of infants of diabetic mothers. *Arch Pediatr Adolesc Med* 1998;152(3):249-54.
16. Webster J, Moore K, McMullan A. Breastfeeding outcomes for women with insulin dependent diabetes. *J Hum Lact* 1995;11(3):195-200.
17. Ferris AM, Dalidowitz CK, Ingardia CM, Reece EA, Fumia FD, Jensen RG, et al. Lactation outcome in insulin-dependent diabetic women. *J Am Diet Assoc* 1988;88(3):317-22.
18. Righard L, Alade MO. Effect of delivery room routines on success of first breast-feed. *Lancet* 1990;336(8723):1105-7.
19. Wright A, Rice S, Wells S. Changing hospital practices to increase the duration of breastfeeding. *Pediatrics* 1996;97(5):669-75.
20. Thorsdottir I, Birgisdottir BE, Johannsdottir IM, Harris DP, Hill J, Steingrimsdottir L, et al. Different beta-casein fractions in Icelandic versus Scandinavian cow's milk may influence diabetogenicity of cow's milk in infancy and explain low incidence of insulin-dependent diabetes mellitus in Iceland. *Pediatrics* 2000;106(4):719-24.

Down syndrome (Trisomy 21)

Summary

Breastmilk is particularly beneficial for infants with Down syndrome. Many of these infants breastfeed without problems, although some experience difficulties.

Definition/cause

Down syndrome is the most common autosomal chromosomal abnormality present in live births, affecting approximately one in 700-800 infants.[1] The individual with Down syndrome has an extra chromosome number 21; hence the anomaly is also known as trisomy 21. In 95% of cases, trisomy 21 due to meiotic nondisjunction is responsible for the syndrome.[2] Translocation Down syndrome accounts for 3-5% of cases, and in a further 3%, mitotic non-disjunction occurs, leading to trisomy 21 mosaicism.[1] Individuals with mosaicism have 46 chromosomes in some cells, and 47 chromosomes in others.

The chance of having a child with Down syndrome increases with maternal age, from 1:2,500 for women under 20 compared to approximately 1:50 for women aged 45. However, because older women have fewer babies than younger women, approximately half the infants with Down syndrome are born to mothers under 35 years of age.[3]

Characteristics

Many infants with trisomy 21 are diagnosed prenatally by amniocentesis or ultrasound. Otherwise, these infants are usually identifiable at birth from a host of characteristic dysmorphic features which include, but are not limited to, a Mongolian slant to the eyes, epicanthal folds, small ears, broad hands with short fingers, excess nuchal skin, large tongue, hypotonia, poor Moro reflex, single transverse palmar crease (simian crease), Brushfield spots (speckling of the iris), and a wide gap between the first and second toes.[2]

Children born with Down syndrome may have additional complications which can include congenital heart defects (in approximately 50% of children), hearing loss (75%), obstructive sleep apnea (50-70%), eye disease (60%) including cataracts (15%), thyroid disease (15%), and gastrointestinal malformations such as duodenal atresia (12%) and Hirschprung disease (<1%).[2] By age three, most children with Down syndrome have retarded growth.[1]

Individuals vary tremendously intellectually and developmentally, but generally their development is slower than in other children (for example, language is delayed, and they may not learn to walk until between 18 and 36 months), and the majority have a below average IQ, which usually ranges from 35-70.[2] Despite the below average IQ, many individuals with Down Syndrome interact well socially,[2] and an enriching home environment and early intervention programs can positively affect the child's development.[2]

Down syndrome and breastfeeding
Benefits of breastmilk

Infants with Down syndrome benefit from breastmilk for a multitude of reasons. Breastmilk reduces infections, and these babies are prone to infections such as otitis media. Breastmilk is also the healthiest option for infants anticipating cardiac surgery or with GI tract complications.

Practical considerations

Traditionally, infants with Down syndrome are described as difficult to feed; breastfeeding can be compromised by hypotonia, sleepiness, and a large tongue. However, one study of 59 babies with Down syndrome recorded that 31 infants had no problem establishing breastfeeding, although severe cardiac anomaly was associated with ineffective sucking.[4] Another study of 44 children with Down syndrome concluded that the condition did not affect the prevalence of breastfeeding when compared with healthy controls.[5]

In terms of positioning, the clutch or football hold can be useful: an upright baby is more likely to remain awake; the mother can see the infant's mouth clearly on the breast, and she can support the head well. The Dancer™ Hand position, which uses the mother's cupped hand to support the infant's chin, can assist a low-tone infant with nursing.

Pillows and rolled cloths can also be used to prop up the head: in fact the whole baby should be well supported, possibly with pillows, otherwise the low tone of the body and extremities tends to pull on the neck and face, drawing the mouth away from the nipple and adversely affecting the latch.

The infant with Down syndrome may be sleepy or passive, and may need to be roused for feeds: weight gain should be carefully monitored. Parents should take advantage of wakeful periods for feeding and for interacting with their infants whenever possible. Sometimes supplemental calories are necessary, especially for those infants who risk slow weight gain as a result of cardiac anomaly, or as a result of a weak suck. Calories can be added to pumped milk in powdered form, or given as a supplemental formula feed where necessary. If the latch is effective, extra nutrition can be given at the breast with a Supplemental Nursing System™ for an infant who nurses weakly (see Breastfeeding aids).

The mother of an infant diagnosed with Down syndrome would be well advised to rent an electric breast pump as soon as possible after the child is born (see Breastfeeding aids); this will provide extra breast stimulation and increase her supply if the infant nurses weakly. It will also prove useful if the infant needs to undergo corrective surgery.

Food for thought

- Kimberly Barbas, BSN, IBCLC is the Lactation Consultant at Children's Hospital in Boston. She frequently works with infants with Down syndrome, many of them with cardiac disease and some with other issues. She says, "I strongly encourage my families to breastfeed. Often they have been told their baby won't be able to breastfeed, or will have trouble gaining weight - I find this to be true far less often than people think: in my experience these babies breastfeed quite well!" Her favorite tips include using leg massage to keep the infants awake, and use of skin to skin holding for tactile stimulation.
- Recent research also points to the possible role of breastmilk in enhancing cognitive ability. Breastmilk contains cholesterol, taurine, and DHA, which are not found in formula, and are important for cell membrane formation in the brain.[6-8] Although studies have not been conducted on children with Down syndrome, one meta-analysis of 20 studies concluded that breastfed children had a 3.16 more IQ points than formula-fed children, even after controlling for all other variables. The same review found that cognitive developmental benefits increased with breastfeeding

duration.[9] Lucas led a multicenter controlled feeding trial among premature infants, (again, these were not infants with Down syndrome) and reported that at 18 months, children who had received breastmilk had improved motor skills, and scored significantly higher on Bayley Developmental Tests, than formula-fed children.[10,11] The same children were reevaluated at 7.5 to 8 years and the breastfed group scored 10 points higher in overall IQ, with an 8.3 IQ point advantage remaining even after adjustment for differences between groups in mother's education and social class.[12] Research also suggests that preterm infants fed breastmilk have faster brainstem maturation than formula-fed infants.[13]

• Dr Jerome Lejeune first reported that individuals with Down syndrome have an extra chromosome in 1959.

Resources

National Down Syndrome Congress
1605 Chantilly Dr., Suite 250
Atlanta, GA 30324-3269
Tel 800/232-6372
Tel 414/633-1555

Association for Children with Down Syndrome
2616 Martin Ave.
Belmore, NY 11710
Tel. 516/221-4700

Foundation for Children with Down Syndrome
17646 N. Cave Creek Rd., Ste 152
Phoenix, AZ 85032
Tel. 612/822-3724
www.ffcwds.org

National Down Syndrome Society
666 Broadway, 8th Fl.,
New York, NY 10012
Tel. 800/221-4602
Tel. 770/604-9500
www.ndss.org

www.nas.com/downsyn: Resources for families affected by Down syndrome.

References

1. Taeusch HW, Avery ME. *Avery's Diseases of the Newborn.* 7th ed. Philadelphia:WB Saunders; 2000:49-52.
2. American Academy of Pediatrics Committee on Genetics. Health Supervision for Children With Down Syndrome. *Pediatrics* 2001;107(2):442-449.
3. Johnson KB, Oski FA. *Oski's Essential Pediatrics.* Philadelphia: Lippincott and Raven; 1997:507-8.
4. Aumonier ME, Cunningham CC. Breast feeding in infants with Down's syndrome. *Child Care Health Dev* 1983;9(5):247-55.
5. Hopman E, Csizmadia CG, Bastiani WF, Engels QM, de Graaf EA, le Cessie S, et al. Eating habits of young children with Down syndrome in The Netherlands: adequate nutrient intakes but delayed introduction of solid food. *J Am Diet Assoc* 1998;98(7):790-4.
6. American Academy of Pediatrics Work Group on Breastfeeding. Breastfeeding and the Use of Human Milk. *Pediatrics* 1997;100(6):1035-1039.
7. Morrow-Tlucak M, Haude RH, Ernhart CB. Breastfeeding and cognitive development in the first 2 years of life. *Soc Sci Med* 1988;26(6):635-9.
8. Wang YS, Wu SY. The effect of exclusive breastfeeding on development and incidence of infection in infants. *J Hum Lact* 1996;12(1):27-30.
9. Anderson JW, Johnstone BM, Remley DT. Breast-feeding and cognitive development: a meta-analysis. *Am J Clin Nutr* 1999;70(4):525-35.
10. Morley R, Cole TJ, Powell R, Lucas A. Mother's choice to provide breast milk and developmental outcome. *Arch Dis Child* 1988;63(11):1382-5.
11. Lucas A, Morley R, Cole TJ, Gore SM, Lucas PJ, Crowle P, et al. Early diet in preterm babies and developmental status at 18 months. *Lancet* 1990;335(8704):1477-81.
12. Lucas A, Morley R, Cole TJ, Lister G, Leeson-Payne C. Breast milk and subsequent intelligence quotient in children born preterm. *Lancet* 1992;339(8788):261-4.
13. Amin SB, Merle KS, Orlando MS, Dalzell LE, Guillet R. Brainstem maturation in premature infants as a function of enteral feeding type. *Pediatrics* 2000;106(2 Pt 1):318-22.

Engorgement

Summary
Frequent breastfeeding is the best solution for the prevention and treatment of engorgement.

Definition/cause
The breasts become firm, heavy, and full of milk at around three days postpartum, when the second stage of lactogenesis begins and the full milk supply 'comes in'. Technically this is postpartum fullness; engorgement is a more uncomfortable experience caused by excessive breast fullness, with possible vascular dilatation. The vessels of the lymphatic system may also become compressed, obstructed, and unable to drain.[1] However, some degree of engorgement is so common that the term is often loosely applied to the entire period of postpartum fullness.

Despite the prevalence of engorgement in industrialized nations at least, little research has been conducted into its cause.[2] One study followed 114 breastfeeding women for 14 days postpartum, and plotted engorgement ratings on a daily basis to provide a visual display of each woman's breast engorgement experience. Four distinct patterns of engorgement were demonstrated: a bell-shaped pattern, a multi-modal pattern, a pattern of intense engorgement, or a pattern of minimal engorgement.[3] Among the same group of women, second time breastfeeding mothers experienced engorgement sooner and more severely than did first time breastfeeding mothers, regardless of the method of birth.[4]

Another study looked at two different methods of breastfeeding: the experimental group breastfed with prolonged emptying of one breast at each feed, and the control group drained both breasts equally at each feed. The experimental group had a lower incidence of breast engorgement in the first week (61.4% versus 74.3%; p 0.02), however there was no significant difference between the two groups in the incidence of mastitis.[5] Although it is commonly believed that increased or prolonged engorgement increases the mother's risk of contracting mastitis, studies do not exist to demonstrate that this is the case. In fact sore and/or cracked nipples is more frequently cited as a predictor of mastitis than is engorgement.[6-8]

Given the lack of research data, clinical experience suggests that optimal breastfeeding management, with early feedings, frequent feedings, and avoidance of supplemental formula help to reduce the incidence and severity of engorgement. Engorgement may also result from excessive pumping, missed feeds, or sudden weaning.

Signs and symptoms

During engorgement the breasts may become large, hard, lumpy, warm, reddened, and painful. Pain and swelling may extend all the way into the axillary region, where mammary tissue also produces milk, in the tail of Spence. Milk may leak from the nipples, or the mother may find it difficult to express milk or latch the baby on because the breasts are swollen. Prolonged engorgement can lead to a drop in milk production, and eventually to atrophy of the milk-secreting cells.[1]

Treatment

The best way to prevent and treat engorgement is to breastfeed more frequently. In the authors' clinical experience, new mothers sometimes 'panic' when the breasts become excessively full, and, especially if the breasts have become so firm that the infant cannot latch, may give the infant a bottle of formula. This approach worsens the situation, as no milk is removed from the breast, which then becomes even more engorged. A true solution requires finding a method to express milk, thereby softening the areola and the breast so the infant can latch and remove milk from the breast.

Hand expression is one way to soften the breast. Treating the breast with warm packs (or warm moist washcloths) prior to hand expression can enhance milk flow. The mother should take the breast in both hands, with the fingers approximately 2 cm behind the nipple. She should push the breast gently in towards the chest wall, then roll the thumb and fingers gently but firmly down towards the nipple. The process should not elicit pain. If the mother stands in a warm shower, milk will drip or flow from the nipples as warm water flows over the breasts, and hand expression will be more effective. Leaning over and submerging both breasts into a sink or dishpan filled with warm water will also allow gravity and warmth to drain milk from the breasts.

Given that many women in western cultures are uncomfortable handling their breasts, too often they and their clinicians may resort to technology. High quality electric breast pumps can effectively treat severe engorgement when used prudently: however, if the baby will latch, there is no reason to use a breast pump - extra pumping will only create extra milk.

If the mother is severely engorged and is unable to latch the baby onto the breast, and if she is unable to soften the breast by hand expression, she can pump for a short period of time with a high quality electric pump (see Breastfeeding aids), until the breast softens enough for the baby to latch on and remove milk more effectively.   If the breasts are severely engorged, even a high quality pump may not prove fully effective the first time it is used.   For the best possible chance of pumping success, the mother should try to relax, use warm compresses or warm water on the breast, then use the pump, on one or both breasts as she prefers.   Sometimes, pumping for short bursts will remove a little milk, then another short burst of pumping later will successfully remove more milk.

To relieve the pain associated with engorgement, the mother can take acetaminophen or ibuprofen, and both warm compresses and cool packs are frequently recommended.   Cool packs (which can be improvised at home with packages of frozen vegetables) will reduce swelling; warmth causes dilation of vessels and is thus useful immediately before a feed.

Many lactation consultants use cabbage leaves to relieve engorgement.   Nikodem reported that women who were treated for engorgement with cabbage leaves at 72 hours postpartum breastfed exclusively, and for longer than untreated women.   However, cabbage leaves did not affect the actual engorgement.[9] Another study found no difference between the use of cabbage leaves when cool or at room temperature, but both groups reported significantly less pain after treatment.[10]   These results are similar to studies done on the effect of cool and warm treatments for engorgement, where both appear advantageous.   Perhaps the beneficial effect is not so much the precise method of treatment, as the act of caring for the mother at this critical time.[9,11]

If engorgement is related to overuse of a breast pump, or to sudden weaning, the mother should be counseled appropriately (see Weaning).

Engorgement and breastfeeding

In the hospital, the new mother often has plenty of help and little milk.   When she arrives home, she may have plenty of milk and little help.   A hungry, crying infant and an emotional, engorged mother are not a good match. Hospital staff should prepare the mother for engorgement before discharge. With time, the body will adjust the amount of milk made to the baby's needs, and engorgement will cease.

Food for thought

* Consistent, accurate breastfeeding information from perinatal staff is crucial in the prevention of severe engorgement.
* On discharge, many hospitals give out diaper bags containing free formula to all mothers. These discharge bags, provided free of charge by formula companies, have been shown to lower exclusive breastfeeding rates, and to shorten breastfeeding duration.[12]

References

1. Lawrence RA, Lawrence RM. *Breastfeeding: A Guide for the Medical Profession*. 5th ed. St. Louis: Mosby, Inc., 1999.
2. Glover R. The engorgement enigma. *Breastfeed Rev* 1998;6(2):31-4.
3. Humenick SS, Hill PD, Anderson MA. Breast engorgement: patterns and selected outcomes. *J Hum Lact* 1994;10(2):87-93.
4. Hill PD, Humenick SS. The occurrence of breast engorgement. *J Hum Lact* 1994;10(2):79-86.
5. Evans K, Evans R, Simmer K. Effect of the method of breast feeding on breast engorgement, mastitis and infantile colic. *Acta Paediatr* 1995;84(8):849-52.
6. Jonsson S, Pulkkinen MO. Mastitis today: incidence, prevention and treatment. *Ann Chir Gynaecol Suppl* 1994;208:84-7.
7. Livingstone V, Stringer LJ. The treatment of Staphyloccocus aureus infected sore nipples: a randomized comparative study. *J Hum Lact* 1999;15(3):241-6.
8. Vogel A, Hutchison BL, Mitchell EA. Mastitis in the first year postpartum. *Birth* 1999;26(4):218-25.
9. Nikodem VC, Danziger D, Gebka N, Gulmezoglu AM, Hofmeyr GJ. Do cabbage leaves prevent breast engorgement? A randomized, controlled study. *Birth* 1993;20(2):61-4.
10. Roberts KL, Reiter M, Schuster D. A comparison of chilled and room temperature cabbage leaves in treating breast engorgement. *J Hum Lact* 1995;11(3):191-4.
11. Riordan J, Auerbach KG. *Breastfeeding and Human Lactation*. Sudbury, MA: Jones and Bartlett, 1999.
12. Frank DA, Wirtz SJ, Sorenson JR, Heeren T. Commercial discharge packs and breast-feeding counseling: effects on infant-feeding practices in a randomized trial. *Pediatrics* 1987;80(6):845-54.

Galactoceles

Summary
Breastfeeding can continue in the presence of a galactocele.

Definition/cause
A galactocele, sometimes called a milk retention cyst, is a benign cyst filled with milky fluid, which can develop in the breast during pregnancy or lactation. Galactoceles are rare. They vary from pea to walnut-size, and are sometimes associated with a plugged milk duct.[1]

Signs and symptoms
A galactocele manifests as a round, mobile lump in the lactating breast. Unlike a plugged duct or infection, the galactocele is usually a source of annoyance rather than of pain. However, one case report records a mother who breastfed several children over the course of 10 years, and experienced constant recurrence of a galactocele in one breast. She suffered several infections and plugged ducts in the same breast.[2]

Treatment
Galactoceles can materialize without apparent cause; they are equally likely to atrophy and resolve without intervention. Some galactoceles, however, do not resolve. Clearly, an accurate diagnosis is important because a breast lump could indicate breast cancer. Fluid can be removed from the galactocele by fine needle aspiration, and analyzed to confirm that the cyst is not malignant;[1] ultrasound can also confirm the diagnosis.[3] Removing the fluid by fine needle aspiration will shrink the cyst, but it often refills with milk. If necessary, the galactocele can be removed by surgery and breastfeeding can continue uninterrupted.

Galactoceles and breastfeeding
No reason exists to interrupt breastfeeding due to the presence of a galactocele.

Food for thought
- Galactoceles containing milky fluid have been recorded in male infants[4,5]

References
1. Novotny DB, Maygarden SJ, Shermer RW, Frable WJ. Fine needle aspiration of benign and malignant breast masses associated with pregnancy. *Acta Cytol* 1991;35(6):676-86.
2. Bevin TH, Pearson CK. Breastfeeding difficulties and a breast abscess associated with a galactocele: a case report. *J Hum Lact* 1993;9(3):177-8.
3. Lawrence RA, Lawrence RM. *Breastfeeding: A Guide for the Medical Profession.* 5th ed. St. Louis: Mosby; 1999:273-274.
4. Boyle M, Lakhoo K, Ramani P. Galactocele in a male infant: case report and review of literature. *Pediatr Pathol* 1993;13(3):305-8.
5. Steiner MM. Bilateral galactocele in a male infant. *J Pediatr* 1967;71(2):240-3.

Galactosemia

Summary
Breastfeeding is contraindicated in an infant with galactosemia.

Definition/cause
Galactosemia is an autosomal recessive inherited disorder of galactose metabolism with an incidence of 1:60,000-1:80:000,[1] occurring equally in males and females. Lactose, the primary carbohydrate in breastmilk, is a disaccharide of glucose and galactose. An infant with classic galactosemia, as discussed here, lacks the enzyme galactose-1-phosphate uridyl transferase, and thus lacks the enzymatic capability to convert galactose to glucose. This causes an abnormal and toxic accumulation of galactose and galactose by-products in the infant.

Signs and symptoms
Symptoms of galactosemia include jaundice, hypoglycemia, vomiting, hepatosplenomegaly, lethargy, bleeding, failure to thrive, and a susceptibility to *Escherichia coli* sepsis. As the disease progresses,

cirrhosis, liver failure, cataracts and mental retardation may develop. If untreated, galactosemia can be lethal.

Treatment

Early diagnosis is crucial, and remarkable progress has been made in the early detection of galactosemia due to mandated newborn metabolic screening in the United States and other countries.

Despite this advance, symptoms may appear before results of the newborn screen are known. If galactosemia is suspected, diagnosis can be confirmed by checking with a Clinitest™ strip (or a similar test) which will identify the non-glucose reducing substance galactose in the urine. To maximize the chance of optimal neurocognitive development, treatment should begin within the first 10 days of life. Once diagnosed, avoidance of lactose and lactose containing products is critical.

Galactosemia and breastfeeding

Breastfeeding is absolutely contraindicated in an infant with classic galactosemia. The infant instead should be fed a lactose-free formula.[2]

Food for thought

• Any newborn diagnosed with a urinary tract infection due to *Escherichia coli* should also have urine screened for galactose to rule out the possibility of galactosemia.

Resources

Parents of Galactosemic Children Inc.
2148 Bryton Dr.
Powell OH 95252
614/840-0473
www.galactosemia.org

References

1. Committee on Genetics: Newborn Screening Fact Sheet. *Pediatrics* 1996;98:473-501.
2. Lawrence RA, Howard CR. Given the Benefits of Breastfeeding, Are There any Contraindications? *Clinics in Perinatology:Clinical Aspects of Human Milk and Lactation.* Wagner CL, Purohit DM eds. June 1999:479-490.

Gonorrhea

Summary

If a mother with untreated gonorrhea gives birth, she should be treated upon diagnosis, and the infant should receive antibiotic therapy. Women with gonorrhea can breastfeed as long as they and their infants are receiving therapy or will imminently be receiving therapy.

Definition/cause

Neisseria gonorrhea is a gram negative bacteria that is transmitted sexually and at birth; humans are the only natural host of the organism.[1] In adults, gonorrhea is a frequently occurring sexually transmitted disease (STD), most commonly seen in individuals between 15 and 24 years of age. High rates of disease are associated with times of low progesterone activity, thus women are most susceptible to contracting gonorrhea during pregnancy and during menses.[1]

Signs and symptoms

In infants the usual site of infection is the eye, but gonococcal disease can also occur as a scalp infection, septic arthritis, bacteremia, meningitis and endocarditis.[1] In adults, the disease causes urethritis in males and cervicitis in females, and can also cause proctitis, pharyngitis, conjunctivitis, perihepatitis, arthritis, meningitis, endocarditis or disseminated disease.

Gonorrhea commonly presents in women with purulent cervical and vaginal discharge, dysuria and/or abnormal menses. Complications include salpingitis and pelvic inflammatory disease, and infertility and ectopic pregnancy may result.

Diagnosis is made by isolation of the organism by culture or by antigen detection using nucleic acid amplification methods. Improved screening technologies mean urine culturing is becoming more frequent.

Treatment

Penicillin was the treatment of choice for many years, but CDC guidelines published in 1993 recommended a change in the first line of treatment for several reasons. The organism was becoming increasingly resistant to penicillin, treatment could effectively be provided by single dose therapy with newer medications, and co-infection with chlamydia was becoming increasingly common. Currently, approximately 50% of US patients with gonorrhea have concurrent chlamydia infections.[1]

Gonorrhea medications and breastfeeding

Because so many women with gonorrhea are co-infected with chlamydia, the present standard is to treat both STDs simultaneously. For gonorrhea, the treatment is a single intramuscular ceftriaxone (125 mg), which is approved by the American Academy of Pediatrics (AAP) for use in breastfeeding mothers, or cefixime (one 400 mg dose by mouth) which would not be expected to cause problems for her healthy breastfeeding infant.[2] This should be given in conjunction with azithromycin (1 gram by mouth x 1) or doxycycline (100mg twice a day for 7 days) to treat chlamydia (see Chlamydia).[3]

The patient should be screened for other sexually transmitted diseases like chlamydia, syphilis, HIV, and hepatitis B, and a history should be taken for herpes or venereal warts. Sexual partners should be treated.

In many countries, standard prenatal care includes a gonorrhea screening test for all pregnant women, and at-risk women are screened again in the third trimester.

An infant born to a GC positive mother is at high risk of having the organism, and antibiotic treatment is recommended. For term newborns, a 125 mg single dose of ceftriaxone, or alternatively a 100 mg single does of cefotaxime, should be administered intravenously or intramuscularly.[3]

Gonorrhea and breastfeeding

Treatment for a woman infected with gonorrhea should begin promptly. When a mother with untreated gonorrhea gives birth, she should be treated immediately upon diagnosis, and the baby should receive prophylactic antibiotic therapy. As long as treatment is initiated or is imminent, the infant born to a mother with gonorrhea can breastfeed. To date there are no reports of the organism being transmitted via breastmilk.[4]

Some reports of infection through poor hygiene exist – the organism can be acquired from exudate or secretions from infected mucous surfaces. Thus the infected mother of a newborn should pay careful attention to personal hygiene.

Food for thought

• In 1881, Dr Carl Sigmund Franz Crede published a paper about preventing gonococcal ophthalmia neonatorum by applying 2% silver nitrate to infant's eyes at birth. This became known as the Crede procedure.[1]

References

1. American Academy of Pediatrics. In Pickering LK, ed. *2000 Red Book: Report of the Committee on Infectious Diseases*. 25th ed. Elk Grove Village, IL: American Academy of Pediatrics; 2000:254-260.
2. Lawrence RA , Lawrence RM. *Breastfeeding: A Guide for the Medical Profession.*5th ed. St Louis:Mosby;1999:579-580.
3. Feigin RD, Cherry, JD eds. *Textbook of Pediatric Infectious Diseases.* 4th ed. Philadelphia: Saunders, 1998:1157-69.
4. Hale TW. *Medications and Mothers' Milk.* 9th ed. Amarillo:Pharmasoft;2000:112.

Group A Streptococcal pharyngitis (Strep throat)

Summary

A woman with strep throat should receive prompt treatment. Her infant should be watched for signs of illness. Breastfeeding is not contraindicated in women with Group A Streptococcal pharyngitis.

Definition/cause

Group A *Streptococcus* (GAS) is a common bacterial cause of acute pharyngitis or 'strep throat', which can affect all age groups, but is most commonly seen in school-aged children, during spring and winter. Spread is usually by infectious droplets, transmitted by close person to person contact. Some individuals remain asymptomatic carriers of the organism, and spread the disease unknowingly. An untreated individual is most infectious during the acute illness and much less contagious after 24-48 hours on appropriate antibiotic treatment. If strep throat remains untreated, suppurative complications can include otitis media, sinusitis, mastoiditis, pharyngeal and retropharyngeal abscesses, and cervical adenitis. Non-suppurative complications include acute glomerulonephritis and acute rheumatic fever.[1]

The second most common site of GAS infections is the skin, where it can cause cellulitis, pyoderma, erysipelas, impetigo and other infections. In children, GAS infection of the skin may complicate a case of chickenpox.

Signs and symptoms

Classically, the illness begins with non-specific complaints of fever, headache, abdominal pain and vomiting. Then the patient develops a sore throat, tonsillar enlargement and erythema, a white-yellow exudate, palatal petechiae, tender anterior cervical nodes, foul breath, a white coated or red tongue, and possibly a scarlatiniform rash, which would be seen with scarlet fever. Characteristically, symptoms occur without signs of an upper respiratory tract infection, and resolve after three to five days in an uncomplicated, untreated case of strep throat. Antibiotic treatment shortens the course of the illness slightly, but more importantly prevents suppurative complications and rheumatic fever.

The infection is rare in children under three years of age, but when acquired it manifests differently, as a syndrome of fever, malaise, lymphadenopathy and purulent rhinorrhea without pharyngitis. Scarlet fever is also rare in children under three due to transplacental passage of antibodies to the toxin.

The gold standard for diagnosis is a culture of the pharynx. Since results of the culture can take time to read, the clinician often also performs the 'quick strep test', which rapidly detects streptococcal antigens, and can be read in minutes.

Treatment

If the 'quick strep' test is positive, the mother will be treated. Penicillin, which is approved by the American Academy of Pediatrics for use in breastfeeding women, is the drug of choice to treat pharyngitis caused by group A streptococcus; erythromycin and cephalosporins (also considered safe for breastfeeding) are alternatives. The affected individual is non-infectious to others approximately 24 hours after antibiotic treatment has begun.[1] The infant of a mother who is infected with strep throat will have been exposed to the condition via contact with the mother, and should thus be watched carefully for potential signs of illness.

Strep throat and breastfeeding
The mother with strep throat can continue to breastfeed, but should take careful precautions around handwashing and handling her infant to avoid possible transmission. She will be most infectious during the acute phase of the disease, and until approximately 24 hours after the antibiotic has taken effect.

Food for thought
• Puppeteer and Sesame Street originator, Jim Henson, died of pneumonia caused by group A *Streptococcus*.
• Group A *Streptococcus* was the cause of puerperal fever, the most common perinatal fatal infection of mothers and infants in the late nineteenth century.[2]

References
1. American Academy of Pediatrics. In Pickering LK, ed. *2000 Red Book: Report of the Committee on Infectious Diseases*. 25th ed. Elk Grove Village, IL: American Academy of Pediatrics; 2000:526-36.
2. Taeusch HW, Avery ME. *Avery's Diseases of the Newborn*. 7th ed. Philadelphia:WB Saunders, 2000:188-90.

Group B *Streptococcus* infection (GBS)

Summary
A mother with Group B *Streptococcus* infection should receive prompt treatment. An infant at high risk of developing GBS should receive prompt treatment. Women and infants with GBS can breastfeed.

Definition/cause

Between 5 and 35% of pregnant women are colonized with group B streptococci, which commonly inhabit the GI and GU tracts, and are a major cause of perinatal bacterial infections in both mother and baby. Although many pregnant women are colonized with GBS, many infants remain uninfected; other infants become colonized but do not become ill, and some infants become infected and become seriously ill. Risk factors for an infant developing GBS disease include prematurity, prolonged rupture of the membranes (>18 hours), a GBS positive mother, and maternal fever ≥ 100.4 degrees, or maternal chorioamnionitis. Transmission from mother to infant occurs shortly before or during delivery.

Signs and symptoms

Maternal GBS infections associated with pregnancy include bacteremia, endometritis, amnionitis, and urinary tract infections.

In infants, GBS infections are defined as 'early onset', in infants under seven days of age, and 'late onset', in infants between seven days and three months of age. Early onset infections usually present within hours of delivery,[1] and can manifest as respiratory distress, apnea, shock, pneumonia, and meningitis. Late onset infections include bacteremia, meningitis or focal infections.[2]

Treatment

If GBS is diagnosed during pregnancy, the mother should be treated with antibiotics.[2] The decision on whether to treat neonates considered to be at high risk for developing a GBS infection is complex, and is calculated according to the number of risk factors present. Factors which can cause a baby to be at 'high risk' for developing GBS disease include prematurity (infant born before 37 weeks gestation), prolonged rupture of the membranes (>18 hours), a GBS positive mother, and maternal fever ≥ 100.4, or maternal chorioamnionitis. A detailed description of the strategy used to calculate the need for treatment is available in *Red Book*.[2] Infants considered to be at risk for GBS have a complete blood count (CBC) and a blood culture drawn as well. Depending on the results of the CBC, the high risk infant may be started on antibiotics before the results of the blood culture are known.

Group B *streptococcus* and breastfeeding

A woman with a GBS infection should be treated promptly, and can breastfeed.   An infant determined to have a high risk of GBS infection should receive appropriate treatment, and can breastfeed. No reason exists to interrupt breastfeeding due to the theoretic risk of infection via breastmilk, because the infected mother and the infant at high risk of developing GBS should already be receiving appropriate antibiotic therapy to combat the documented threat of perinatal transmission.

References

1.   Taeusch HW, Avery ME.   *Avery's Diseases of the Newborn.*   7th ed. Philadelphia: WB Saunders; 2000:188-90.
2.   American Academy of Pediatrics.   In:Pickering LK, ed.   *2000 Red Book: Report of the Committee on Infectious Diseases.*   25th ed.   Elk Grove Village, IL:Amercian Academy of Pediatrics 2000:537-544.

Hepatitis A

Summary

The mother with hepatitis A can breastfeed.

Definition/cause

Hepatitis A is a viral infection of the liver, caused by the RNA-containing hepatitis A virus (HAV).   It is most commonly transmitted person to person via the fecal oral route, and sources of infection include childcare centers, contaminated drinking water, or foods such as shellfish that have been exposed to human sewerage. Hepatitis A is an acute, self-limited illness, which usually lasts several weeks.   Unlike the more aggressive hepatitis B, it does not cause chronic infection, and rarely develops into overwhelming hepatitis.

The spread of HAV can be prevented by thorough handwashing and effective sanitation.   Anti-HAV antibodies developed during an infection guarantee lifetime immunity to the disease.

Signs and symptoms
Symptoms of hepatitis A in adults include fever, jaundice, malaise, constipation, nausea, vomiting, abdominal pain, anorexia, and dark colored urine.   The disease is often subclinical in the infant and child,[1] or can present as a non-specific illness without jaundice.

Treatment
Prevention is the best strategy: once acquired, the only treatment is symptomatic – rest and maintenance of adequate hydration. Hepatitis A vaccines are available, although not for children under two years of age.[2] Vaccination is recommended when visiting areas where hepatitis A is endemic, and for high-risk segments of the population, such as patients with chronic liver disease.   An intramuscular shot of immune globulin is between 80 and 90% effective at preventing systemic development of the disease in exposed adults.[3]

Hepatitis A and breastfeeding
For numerous reasons, maternal hepatitis A infection is of less concern than infections associated with other hepatitis viruses. Maternal HAV infection during pregnancy and around the time of birth does not appear to increase the infant's risk of developing hepatitis A.[3] Incidences of vertical transmission are rare,[4] and it does not appear that HAV is transmitted in breastmilk.[3] Finally, acquisition of the disease by infants is often sub-clinical, self-limited, and not associated with a chronic carrier state, or with subsequent, more serious liver disease.

Whether the disease occurs in the mother of a newborn or of an older infant, the mother should practice careful hygiene to prevent a possible infection.   Consideration may be given to prophylactically treating the infant with immune globulin.

In all scenarios, the mother with hepatitis A can breastfeed.

References
1.   Lawrence RA, Lawrence RM.   Breastfeeding: A Guide for the Medical Profession.   5th ed.   St. Louis:Mosby;1999:579-80.
2.   Harris N, Edwards K.   A progress report on hepatitis A vaccination. *Cont Peds* 1998;15(12):64-69.
3.   American Academy of Pediatrics.   In Pickering LK, ed. *2000 Red Book: Report of the Committee on Infectious Diseases.*   25th ed.   Elk

Grove Village, IL: American Academy of Pediatrics; 2000:280-89.
4. Watson JC, Fleming DW, Borella AJ, Olcott ES, Conrad RE, Baron RC. Vertical transmission of hepatitis A resulting in an outbreak in a neonatal intensive care unit. *J Infect Dis* 1993;167(3):567-71.

Hepatitis B

Summary
The mother with hepatitis B can breastfeed.

Definition/cause
Hepatitis B is a viral infection of the liver caused by the DNA-containing hepatitis B virus (HBV). The virus is transmitted predominantly by the parenteral route via the exchange of infected blood or bodily fluids. Common modes of transmission are perinatal transmission, sexual transmission, percutaneous transmission (such as a needle stick or shared needles), and household contact (for example, a shared toothbrush).

Vertical (mother to infant) transmission of hepatitis B during the perinatal period is most commonly by blood contact during birth. In many countries women are screened for the hepatitis B surface antigen (HBsAg) during pregnancy, and a mother who tests positive for HBsAg is considered infected and at risk of transmitting the virus to her infant at birth. A mother who is positive with the hepatitis Be antigen (HBeAg) is highly infectious, and her risk of transmitting the illness to the neonate at birth without treatment is 70-90%.[1]

Hepatitis B is particularly concerning because individuals who contract the acute infection are at risk of becoming chronic HBV carriers. Chronic infection is associated with chronic hepatitis, cirrhosis, and hepatocellular carcinoma (HCC). The younger the age of infection, the greater the chance of becoming a chronic carrier. Ninety percent of infants infected perinatally develop chronic infection, compared to 30% of children infected between the ages of 1 and 5 years, and to 10% of individuals infected as adults.[2] Hepatitis B causes death from liver disease in up to 25% of those infected at birth.[3]

Signs and symptoms

The range of presentation of hepatitis B varies widely, from asymptomatic seroconversion to fulminate hepatitis. Clinical symptoms include anorexia, nausea, malaise, vomiting, abdominal pain, fever, headache, arthritis, arthralgias, macular rash and jaundice, though only one-quarter of those with clinical symptoms will have jaundice.[3] Sub acute, non-specific illness characterized, for example, by mild nausea and general malaise, is more common in children than in adults.

Treatment

There is no specific treatment for acute hepatitis B. Symptomatic treatment includes rest, hydration and close monitoring for potential chronic symptoms.

The hepatitis B vaccine provides immunity to HBV, and will also prevent development of the disease after exposure (but not once infected). Hepatitis B immune globulin (HBIG) offers temporary protection in specific circumstances after exposure to HBV.[2]

Hepatitis B and breastfeeding

According to the American Academy of Pediatrics (AAP) "Studies...have indicated that breastfeeding by HbsAg-positive women does not increase significantly the risk of infection among their infants."[2] However, due to the high risk of vertical transmission, the likelihood of an infant developing chronic carrier status, and the potentially serious sequela from long term infection, clear recommendations for all HBV positive mothers have been developed.[2]

If the mother tests HbsAg positive, the newborn should receive HBIG (0.5cc IM) and the hepatitis B vaccine within 12 hours of birth. The initial vaccination series needs to be followed up with further shots at two and six months of age, and the infant should be checked between one to three months after completion of vaccination series for the presence of antibodies to Hepatitis B surface antigen (anti Hbs).

If the mother's HBsAg status is unknown, she should be tested as soon as possible after the infant's birth, and her newborn should receive the hepatitis B vaccine within 12 hours of birth. If the mother tests positive, HBIG should also be given within seven days of birth, and the vaccination series should be completed at two and six months; if she tests negative, the vaccination series should be followed up at two months and then between 6-18 months.

According to the AAP's most recent guidelines, "In the United States, infants born to known HbsAg-positive women should receive HBIG and hepatitis B virus vaccine, effectively eliminating any theoretical risk of transmission through breastfeeding. There is no need to delay initiation of breastfeeding until after the infant is immunized."[2]

Food for thought

- 90% of healthy adults develop protective antibodies from the three shot hepatitis B series, however some individuals may never develop antibodies.[3]

- In highly endemic hepatitis B areas, which include China, Southeast Asia, Africa, most Pacific Islands, the Amazon Basin, Eastern Europe, and the Middle East, there is a 5-15% carrier rate. In low endemic areas (United States, Western Europe, Australia) there is a 0.1-0.5% carrier rate. In moderate endemic areas (other areas of the world) the carrier rate is 1-4%.[3]

- The hepatitis B virus is also known as the Dane Particle.

References

1. Nowicki MJ, Balistreri WF.   Hepatitis A to E: Building up the alphabet. *Contemporary Pediatrics* 1992;9(11):118-128.
2. American Academy of Pediatrics. In: Pickering LK, ed. *2000 Red Book: Report of the Committee on Infectious Diseases.* 25th ed. Elk Grove Village, IL: American Academy of Pediatrics;2000:100 & 289-302.
3. *Hepatitis B Coalition.* 1573 Selby Ave. Suite 229, St. Paul, MN 55104.

Hepatitis C

Summary
Maternal hepatitis C infection is not a contraindication for breastfeeding.

Definition/cause

Hepatitis C is a viral infection of the liver caused by the RNA-containing hepatitis C virus (HCV). An individual who tests positives for either IgG antibodies to hepatitis C antigens (anti-HCV), or for hepatitis C RNA virus particles (HCV- RNA) is considered infected.

The major mode of transmission is via direct exposure to infected blood or blood products, thus intravenous drug users, hemophiliacs who have received numerous blood transfusions, and individuals with repeated per cutaneous exposure, such as hemodialysis patients, are particularly at risk.[1] The current possibility of acquiring HCV from a blood transfusion in the US is approximately 0.1%:[1] donated blood is thoroughly screened, but currently available serological assays fail to detect HCV antibodies in 5% of cases. In addition, some blood is donated in the period of infection preceding the appearance of antibodies.[1]

Other, less common modes of transmission are by perinatal, sexual, occupational, and household routes. Vertical transmission of hepatitis C occurs in about 5% of carrier mothers,[2] and the higher the mother's viral load, the greater the risk of transmission.[3] If the mother is co-infected with HIV, the rate of vertical transmission of hepatitis C also increases.[4] Infants born to an infected mother will carry maternal anti-HCV antibodies; if they still test positive for anti-HCV antibodies at one year of age, by which time maternal antibodies will have disappeared, they are considered HCV infected.

Signs and symptoms

The clinical course of the disease is usually mild or asymptomatic. When symptoms occur they are often vague and include fatigue, malaise, nausea, anorexia, arthralgia and weight loss. Jaundice occurs in only 25% of cases.[5]

Most pediatric patients with HCV are asymptomatic. However, as with hepatitis B, hepatitis C sufferers have a high risk (75-85%) of becoming chronically infected,[1] which leads to chronic hepatitis in about 70% of cases and to cirrhosis in about 20%.[1] Hepatocellular carcinoma (HCC) can also result from chronic infection; the rate is unknown.

HCV undergoes a high rate of mutation during replication, making it difficult for the body to mount an effective immune response.

Treatment

Interferon, alone or in combination with ribavirin, is approved for use in patients over 18, and has been used with some success to treat adults with chronic HCV infection.[1] However, immune globulin is not effective in preventing infection or disease, and to date there is no hepatitis C vaccine.[2]

Hepatitis C medications and breastfeeding

Little is known about the transfer of interferons into human milk, however their large molecular weight is likely to limit such transfer.   A case study of one patient treated with a massive intravenous dose of 30 million IU found that the amount of interferon transferred into human milk was only minimal (1551 IU/mL) when compared to control milk (1249 IU/mL).[6]   The long term use of ribavirin however is more problematic.   The breastfeeding infant who is exposed to ribavirin over a 6 to 12 month period is at risk of accumulating high levels of the medication, and caution is recommended.[7]

Hepatitis C and breastfeeding

Hepatitis C infection in the mother is not considered a contraindication for breastfeeding.[2,8]   Studies have found both anti-HCV and HCV-RNA in colostrum and breastmilk,[4,9] but no cases of hepatitis C infection via breastmilk have been identified.[1,4,9] Several studies specifically examined the role of breastmilk in hepatitis C transmission.   One followed 15 HCV positive mothers, 11 of whom breastfed.   Although both anti-HCV antibody and HCV- ribonucleic acid were present in colostrum samples, none of the breastfed babies developed hepatitis C infection.[9]   Another study followed 76 HCV positive women who breastfed, and found that only one baby developed hepatitis C, which was identified at one month of age and was not believed to be associated with breastfeeding.[10]

Food for thought

- The hepatitis C virus was discovered in 1989.   Prior to that time, it probably caused many cases of non-A, non-B hepatitis.[5]
- Since 1990, blood and blood products used in the US have been

screened for hepatitis C.[2]

- Almost 4,000,000 Americans have been infected with hepatitis C.[8]
- In adults, chronic HCV infection is the most common cause of liver transplantation in the US.[2]

Resources
Centers for Disease Control:
http://www.cdc.gov/ncidod/diseases/hepatitis/resource/hepcprev.htm #4
Tel. 888/4-HEP-CDC

References
1. American Academy of Pediatrics.   In Pickering LK, ed. *2000 Red Book: Report of the Committee on Infectious Diseases.* 25th ed. Elk Grove Village, IL: American Academy of Pediatrics;2000:302-306.
2. American Academy of Pediatrics Committee on Infectious Disease: Hepatitis C virus infection.   *Pediatrics* 1998;101(3):481-485.
3. Ohto H, Terazawa S, Sasaki N, al e. Transmission of hepatitis C virus from mother to infants. *N Engl J Med* 1994;330:744.
4. Zanetti AR, Tanzi E, Paccagnini S, Principi N, Pizzocolo G, Caccamo ML, et al.   Mother-to-infant transmission of hepatitis C virus. Lombardy Study Group on Vertical HCV Transmission. *Lancet* 1995;345(8945):289-91.
5. Zellos A, Scwarz B. What's the latest on hepatitis C? *Contemporary Pediatrics* 1998;15(4):39-58.
6. Kumar AR, Hale TW, Mock RE. Transfer of interferon alfa into human breast milk. *J Hum Lact* 2000;16(3):226-8.
7. Hale TW.   *Medications and Mothers' Milk.*   9th ed. Amarillo: Pharmasoft Publishing, 2000:580-81.
8. Centers for Disease Control and Prevention, National Center for Infectious Diseases, Division of Viral and Rickettsial Diseases, Hepatitis Branch 2000.
9. Lin HH, Kao JH, Hsu HY, Ni YH, Chang MH, Huang SC, et al. Absence of infection in breast-fed infants born to hepatitis C virus-infected mothers.   *J Pediatr* 1995;126(4):589-91.
10. Polywka S, Schroter M, Feucht HH, Zollner B, Laufs R. Low risk of vertical transmission of hepatitis C virus by breast milk.   *Clin Infect Dis* 1999;29(5):1327-9.

Herpes simplex virus

Summary

The mother with herpes simplex virus can breastfeed, unless she has active lesions near the nipple or areola. If she has active lesions, she should postpone breastfeeding on the affected breast/s until they are healed.

Definition/cause

The herpes simplex virus causes mucocutaneous and systemic disease in all age groups. As a rule of thumb, herpes simplex virus type 1 (HSV-1) is most commonly associated with face and skin lesions above the waist; and herpes simplex virus type 2 (HSV-2) is usually associated with genital and skin lesions below the waist. However, either virus may be found in either site.

In children, the most common herpes simplex induced primary infection is gingivostomatitis, most commonly caused by HSV-1.

HSV-2 is the most common cause of the potentially fatal neonatal herpes infection. Herpes simplex infection can also be responsible for premature birth.

Both herpes simplex viruses are members of the herpesvirus family that includes varicella-zoster virus, cytomegalovirus, Ebstein-Barr virus, and human herpes virus types 6, 7 and 8. As with some other members of the herpes virus family, after a primary infection, the herpes simplex virus enters a latent phase, resting dormant in nerve root ganglia. Recurrent infection, causing milder disease than the primary infection, occurs when the virus is reactivated.

Transmission is by infected bodily fluids or by direct contact with the lesions; in approximately 85% of neonates the disease is acquired by passage through an infected birth canal. The risk of HSV infection from a vaginal birth to a mother with active lesions due to primary infection is 33-50%; a cesarean birth may thus be indicated, depending on when the membranes ruptured. The risk of infection decreases to 0-5% if symptoms are due to a reactivation of the latent virus.[1]

Signs and symptoms

In sexually active adolescents and adults, the disease is

commonly transmitted sexually, and presents as genital herpes due to HSV-2. Both primary disease and reactivation of the virus result in painful vesicular and ulcerative lesions in the genital area.

Gingivostomatitis in children peaks between the ages of six months and three years, causing fever, irritability, and refusal to eat or drink, due to mouth sores located more in the anterior portion than posterior portion of the mouth. Reactivation of the virus results in cold sores.

Herpes simplex infection in the neonate can cause serious illness or death, particularly in the disseminated form, and survivors often have neurological and/or ocular sequela. The infection may be present at birth, or may appear as late as six weeks of age.[1] It can present in many ways: 40% of the time it manifests as an infection of the skin, eye and mucous membranes; 35% of the time it appears as localized, central nervous system disease (encephalitis) and in 25% of cases it is a disseminated disease involving many organs, especially the liver (hepatitis) and lung (pneumonia).[1] The disseminated and CNS versions may or may not be associated with skin lesions.[1]

Treatment

Acyclovir, which is approved by the American Academy of Pediatrics for use in breastfeeding mothers, is the prime therapy for HSV infection in adults, children and infants.[2] The adult should be screened for other sexually transmitted diseases like chlamydia, gonorrhea, syphilis, HIV, and hepatitis B, and a history should be taken for venereal warts.

Herpes simplex virus and breastfeeding

Breastfeeding is not contraindicated in the mother with herpes, unless she has active near the nipple, in which case she should not breastfeed from the affected breast until the lesions are fully healed. Covering of lesions on other areas of the breast is recommended while breastfeeding. Direct contact with active lesions can cause infection,[3] and the mother should practice good handwashing to eliminate the risk of infection from active lesions in other sites.

Food for thought

• In rare cases, the herpes simplex virus can be transmitted from the child's mouth to the mother's breast. In one case report, a 15 month old with gingivostomatitis transmitted symptomatic herpes infection to both maternal nipples through breastfeeding.[4]

References
1. American Academy of Pediatrics. In: Pickering LK. ed. *2000 Red Book: Report of the Committee on Infectious Diseases.* 25th ed. Elk Grove Village, IL: American Academy of Pediatrics;2000:309-318.
2. Hale TW. *Clinical Therapy in Breastfeeding Patients.* Amarillo:Pharmasoft Publishing, 1999:92.
3. Sullivam-Bolyai JZ, Fife KH, Jacobs RF, al e. Disseminated neonatal herpes simplex virus type 1 from a maternal breast lesion. *Pediatrics* 1983;71:455.
4. Sealander JY, Kerr CP. Herpes simplex of the nipple: infant-to-mother transmission. *Am Fam Physician* 1989;39(3):111-3.

Human immunodeficiency virus (HIV)

Summary
Breastfeeding is contraindicated in HIV infected women in nations where safe alternative feeding methods are available. In nations where clean water is lacking, and infectious diseases and malnutrition pose a high mortality risk for infants and children, the World Health Organization recommends women breastfeed irrespective of HIV status.

Definition/cause

HIV infection is caused by cytopathic human retroviruses, human immunodeficiency virus type 1 (HIV-1), and less commonly, by human immunodeficiency virus type 2 (HIV-2).[1] HIV infection causes a wide range of diseases, of which AIDS is the most severe manifestation. The virus persists in the infected person for life.

HIV has been isolated from many bodily fluids, but only blood, semen, cervicovaginal secretions, and human milk have been implicated in the transmission of infection. Transmission occurs primarily by sexual contact. The second most common method of infection is by per cutaneous or mucous membrane contact with infected blood or secretions. Vertical transmission, from mother to infant around birth, accounts for an estimated 13-39% of cases, and high maternal viral load is the major risk factor for both intra-uterine and intra-partum mother-to-child transmission.[2] In the non-breastfeeding dyad, of those infants infected, one-third are infected intrauterine, and two thirds are infected during delivery.[3] Finally, breastfeeding has been implicated as a mode of infection, although studies disagree on the rate of transmission via breastmilk.

HIV and breastfeeding
Risk of HIV infection via breastmilk

A study published in *JAMA* reviewed 672 infants who were HIV-negative at birth, born to HIV-infected women who had not received antiretroviral drugs during or after pregnancy. Forty-seven children became HIV-infected while breastfeeding, and the cumulative infection rate while breastfeeding, from month one to the end of months five, 11, 17, and 23, was 3.5%, 7.0%, 8.9%, and 10.3%, respectively. Incidence per month was 0.7% between one and five months, 0.6% between six and 11 months, and 0.3% between 12 and 17 months.[4]

Another study conducted in South Africa and published in *Lancet* found that at three months of age, 18.8% of 156 never-breastfed children were estimated to be HIV-1 infected, compared with 21.3% of 393 breastfed children. The estimated proportion of infants HIV-1 infected by three months (14.6%) was significantly lower for those exclusively breastfed than in those who received mixed feeding (24.1%), and was comparable to the risk of not breastfeeding. The authors concluded, "If our findings are confirmed, exclusive breastfeeding may offer HIV-1- infected women in developing countries an affordable, culturally acceptable, and effective means of reducing mother-to-child transmission of HIV-1 while maintaining the overwhelming benefits of breastfeeding."[5]

Factors associated with breastfeeding and HIV transmission

Factors which appear to increase the risk of HIV transmission via breastfeeding include maternal nipple lesions, mastitis, reduced maternal CD4 cell count, and maternal seroconversion while breastfeeding.[6]

Trials of short-course zidovudine regimens have effectively reduced vertical transmission, in breastfeeding and non-breastfeeding populations. Nevirapine has been shown to be significantly more effective than short course zidovudine regimens in breastfeeding populations.[2]

Current guidelines of the World Health Organization (WHO), United Nations Children's Fund (UNICEF), and the Joint Nations Programme on HIV/AIDS (UNAIDS):

When children born to women living with HIV can be ensured uninterrupted access to nutritionally adequate breastmilk substitutes that are safely prepared and fed to them, they are at less risk of illness and death if they are not breastfed. However, when these conditions are not fulfilled, in particular in an environment where infectious diseases and malnutrition are the primary causes of death during infancy, artificial feeding substantially increases children's risk of illness and death. In most countries, policy must cover a range of socioeconomic conditions, and the aim should be to promote and protect breastfeeding for the majority of women while offering as much choice as possible to women who are HIV positive, enabling them to decide what is most appropriate for their circumstances and supporting them in their choice.[7]

Food for thought
- HIV was first discovered in breastmilk in 1985.[8]

Resources
CDC National AIDS Hotline
American Society Health Assn.
PO Box 13827
Research Triangle Park, NC 27709
Tel. 800/342-2437
Tel. 800/344-7432 (Spanish)
www.ashastd.org

National Pediatric & Family HIV Resource Center
30 Bergen St. - ADMC - 4
Newark, NJ 07107
Tel. 800/362-0071
Tel. 973/972-0410
www.wdcnet.com/pedsaids

References
1. American Academy of Pediatrics. In Pickering LK, ed. *2000 Red Book: Report of the Committee on Infectious Diseases.* 25th ed. Elk Grove Village, IL: American Academy of Pediatrics; 2000:325-50.
2. Thorne C, Newell ML. Epidemiology of HIV infection in the newborn. *Early Hum Dev* 2000;58(1):1-16.
3. Weinberg GA. The Dilemma of Postnatal Mother-to-Child Transmission of HIV: To Breastfeed or Not? *Birth* 2000;27(3):199-205.
4. Miotti PG, Taha TE, Kumwenda NI, Broadhead R, Mtimavalye LA, Van der Hoeven L, et al. HIV transmission through breastfeeding: a study in Malawi. *JAMA* 1999;282(8):744-9.
5. Coutsoudis A, Pillay K, Spooner E, Kuhn L, Coovadia HM. Influence of infant-feeding patterns on early mother-to-child transmission of HIV-1 in Durban, South Africa: a prospective cohort study. South African Vitamin A Study Group. *Lancet* 1999;354(9177):471-6.
6. Embree JE, Njenga S, Datta P, Nagelkerke NJ, Ndinya-Achola JO, Mohammed Z, et al. Risk factors for postnatal mother-child transmission of HIV-1. *Aids* 2000;14(16):2535-41.
7. World Health Organization. HIV and Infant Feeding: Guidelines for Decision-makers. Publication Nos. WHO/FRH/NUT98.1, UNAIDS/98.3, UNICEF/PD/NUT/(J) 98.1. Geneva: World Health Organization, 1998.
8. Morrison P. HIV and infant feeding: to breastfeed or not to breastfeed: the dilemma of competing risks. Part 1. *Breastfeed Rev* 1999;7(2):5-13.

Hydrocephalus

Summary
A baby with hydrocephalus can breastfeed or receive breastmilk.

Definition/cause

Hydrocephalus, which can be a congenital or an acquired disorder, occurs when an excessive amount of cerebrospinal fluid (CSF) is present in the cerebral ventricles, causing increased pressure within the ventricular system.

CSF is made primarily by the choroid plexus, located in the lateral, third and fourth ventricles of the brain. Under normal circumstances, CSF flows via a pressure gradient from the lateral ventricles through the foramina of Monro into the third ventricle, on through the aqueduct of Sylvius into the fourth ventricle, then exits via foramina (Luschka and Mgendie) into the cisterns at the base of the brain. It then circulates posteriorly through the cistern system and over the cerebral hemispheres, and is absorbed by the arachnoid villi into venous channels of the sagittal sinus. The total volume of CSF is about 50 mL in an infant and 150 mL in an adult; 25% of this is within the ventricular system. CSF turns over 3-4 times per day.[1] In most cases, hydrocephalus involves impaired absorption of CSF due either to a block or a defect in absorption, not an overproduction.

In *noncommunicating or obstructive hydrocephalus,* the block is within the ventricular system. In *communicating hydrocephalus*, the block is outside the ventricular system. The most frequent cause of noncommunicating or obstructive hydrocephalus is aqueductal stenosis. A common cause of communicating hydrocephalus is subarachnoid hemorrhage. Approximately one third of premature infants under 1500g develop some type of intraventricular hemorrhage.

Other causes of hydrocephalus can include congenital abnormalities like meningomyelocele (Arnold-Chiari malformation), Dandy-Walker malformation, chromosomal abnormalities; traumatic deliveries, and intrauterine infections such as rubella, cytomegalovirus, toxoplasmosis, and syphilis.

Complications of meningitis, tumors, aneurysm, and trauma can also result in hydrocephalus.

Signs and symptoms

In young children, prior to fusing of the sutures, hydrocephalus can manifest as excessive head growth, bulging anterior fontanelle, and dilated scalp veins. In older children, adolescents, and adults,

hydrocephalus can cause headaches, early morning vomiting, and irritability. Other symptoms include third and sixth cranial nerve deficits (diplopia), papilledema, and 'sun setting sign': paralysis of upper gaze with downward rolling of the eyeballs so the sclera are visible above the iris, and hyperreflexia. Diagnosis is made by CAT scan or MRI.
Hydrocephalus is often associated with cognitive disabilities.

Treatment

The aim of therapy is to relieve intracranial pressure, and the most frequent treatment is the surgical insertion of an extracranial shunt. This relieves the pressure, but is not a cure. The commonly used ventriculoperitoneal shunt runs from the ventricular system, and is tunneled under the skin on the side of the head, neck, and trunk, into the peritoneal cavity. There the CSF is reabsorbed. The less frequently used ventriculoatrial shunt drains into the right atrium; the ventriculopleural shunt drains to the pleural space.

Hydrocephalus and breastfeeding

If the infant is able to suckle, the mother should be encouraged to breastfeed her infant. Mothers are understandably nervous about handling a baby who has recently undergone surgery, and has a shunt incision on the head. The clinician can assist the mother to find a position which involves supporting the child's shoulders and upper back, and keeps her hands away from the incision; accidentally touching the incision while feeding can cause pain and breast refusal. As in other similar situations, breastfeeding the child with a birth anomaly can help to normalize the situation for the mother and help her to connect with her baby.

Food for thought

• Hydrocephalus is also known as water on the brain.

Resources

Hydrocephalus Association
879 Market St., Ste. 705
San Francisco, CA 94102
Tel. 888/598-3789

www.hydroassoc.org

National Hydrocephalus Foundation
12413 Centralia Rd.
Lakewood, CA 90715-1623
Tel. 888/260-1789
Tel. 562/402-3523
www.geocities.com/HOTSPRINGS/villa/2300

References

1. McMillan JA, DeAngelis CD, Feigin RD, Warshaw JB eds. *Oski's Pediatrics:Principles and Practice.* 3rd ed. Philadelphia:Lippincourt Williams and Wilkins;1999:1906-8.

Hyperbilirubinemia of the term newborn

Summary

"The American Academy of Pediatrics discourages the interruption of breast-feeding in healthy term newborns and encourages continued and frequent breast-feeding (at least eight to ten times every 24 hours). Supplementing nursing with water or dextrose water does not lower the bilirubin level in jaundiced, healthy, breast-feeding infants."[1] Beyond this basic guideline, the AAP presents alternative options for treatment of persistent early onset jaundice in the breastfed term newborn (see below).

Definition/cause

Bilirubin is a product of heme degradation; heme sources include red blood cells, muscle myoglobin, erythropoiesis, cytochromes and other heme proteins. Unconjugated bilirubin is a fat soluble compound and thus can cross into the brain via the blood brain barrier. In the blood stream, bilirubin is transported bound to albumin. Upon arrival at the liver, there is a rapid flux of bilirubin into liver cells where it is bound to ligandin proteins. In the liver cells, the enzyme glucuronyl transferase facilitates the conjugation of bilirubin with glucuronic acid. Now water soluble as conjugated bilirubin, it leaves the liver and is excreted into the gastrointestinal tract.   There it is hydrogenated, producing urobilinogens which are excreted in feces or reabsorbed and excreted in urine.   Conjugated bilirubin in the gut, which is not hydrogenated, can be converted back to unconjugated bilirubin by bacteria, and this unconjugated bilirubin can be reabsorbed into the blood stream via the enterohepatic circulation.   Meconium is loaded with unconjugated bilirubin; the longer it remains in the gut, the more likely it is that enterohepatic circulation will occur.   Unlike formula, colostrum has a laxative effect on the gut, which helps to remove meconium more quickly.

Hyperbilirubinemia (an elevated bilirubin in comparison with the normal adult) is universally present in newborns.   Annually, 60% of the 4,000,000 infants born in the United States become clinically jaundiced in the first days of life due to an elevation of unconjugated bilirubin.[1]   This normal process is referred to as "physiologic jaundice of the newborn."

Healthy term infants produce more bilirubin (8 mg/kg/day) than adults (3-4 mg/kg/day).[2]   Most of the newborn bilirubin comes from red blood cells.   The newborn is born with a high load of red blood cells, having a normal hematocrit of 45-65.   These red blood cells have a shorter life span (90 days) than adult red blood cells (120 days).   In utero, fetal unconjugated bilirubin is handled by the placenta and the maternal liver.   The newborn's liver is immature in its ability to metabolize bilirubin, with a decreased rate of hepatic uptake and a decreased rate of conjugation in the newborn compared to the adult.   In addition, there is an increase in enterohepatic circulation of bilirubin in the newborn.   *The combination of these normal physiologic factors causes physiologic jaundice, which is benign and self limited, and usually resolves without treatment by the end of the first week of life.*

Early onset jaundice or 'lack of breastfeeding jaundice' is caused by an exaggeration of this normal process.   Akin to adult starvation jaundice, neonatal jaundice can be caused by insufficient intake of fluid, calories, or milk.   In the breastfed neonate, hyperbilirubinemia is often associated with lack of frequent feeds (fewer than eight in 24 hours), a weight loss greater than 7%, lack of evidence of the mother's milk coming in, fewer than three bowel movements in 24 hours, and a sleepy, undemanding baby.

> ## Treatment Options for Jaundiced Breast-Fed Infants[1]
> - Observe
> - Continue breast-feeding; administer phototherapy
> - Supplement breast-feeding with formula with or without phototherapy
> - Interrupt breast-feeding; substitute formula
> - Interrupt breast-feeding; substitute formula; administer phototherapy"

In the breastfeeding dyad, poor hospital practices, a lack of breastfeeding knowledge among clinicians, and a lack of support for breastfeeding women often lead to infrequent, ineffective breastfeeding in the early days postpartum. With a low intake of breastmilk, the ineffectively breastfed baby is more vulnerable to high bilirubin levels, hence the term, "lack of breastfeeding jaundice".

Pathological issues and risks associated with hyperbilirubinemia of the newborn, which are distinct from feeding issues, can include hemolytic disease of the newborn (ABO or Rh incompatibility), pyruvate kinase deficiency, hereditary spherocytosis, sepsis, being the infant of a diabetic mother (IDM), hypothyroidism, Lucey-Driscoll Syndrome, and Crigler Najjar syndrome.   An intestinal obstruction, or swallowing of maternal blood during delivery, can also lead to hyperbilirubinemia. (Note: the AAP Guidelines[1] do not apply to pathological issues; they are specifically to the treatment of otherwise healthy newborns).

Signs and symptoms

Lack of breastmilk jaundice usually develops over the first few days of life. When bilirubin levels exceed 5 mg/dl, the infant's skin begins to appear yellow-tinged.[3] Jaundice progresses from the head to the toes ('cephalocaudal progression'); the level of unconjugated bilirubin can be roughly estimated by observing the spread of the yellow coloring from the head and neck (4-8 mg/dL), to the upper (5-12 mg/dL) then lower trunk and thighs (8-16 mg/dL), to the arms and lower legs (11-18 mg/dL). If pigmentation is visible on the palms and soles, bilirubin levels usually exceed 15 mg/dL.[4]

High circulating levels of unconjugated bilirubin are toxic to the central nervous system, especially the basal ganglia. Kernicterus (a pathologic finding of bilirubin pigment deposition in the brain) is a dangerous condition resulting from excessively high bilirubin levels. Kernicterus causes brain encephalopathy, which can manifest as lethargy, change in muscle tone, subtle changes in the brainstem audio evoked response (BAER), and as opisthotonos, extensor rigidity, tremors, ataxic gait, oculomotor paralysis, and hearing loss.

Treatment

The association between early onset jaundice and breastfeeding has led to many erroneous myths and practices. The temporary interruption of breastfeeding as part of the management of early onset hyperbilirubinemia may imply to the parents that breastmilk is the cause, whereas in reality, the problem is usually caused by a *lack* of breastmilk. The picture is further complicated and confused by the fact that in *late onset jaundice* or *breastmilk jaundice*, something in the milk appears to trigger a genetic predisposition for hyperbilirubinemia in certain infants. (See Late onset hyperbilirubinemia.)

According to Dr. Frank Oski, "There is probably no myth that drives clinical practice more than the widespread belief that a serum bilirubin value of 20 mg/dL is capable of producing brain damage in a term infant."[5] Oski coined the term "vigintiphobia" to describe this phenomenon. In order to offset some of the fear surrounding hyperbilirubinemia, Oski offered his own set of guidelines two years prior to the AAP practice parameter. He advised, "In the healthy term infant with no evidence of hemolytic disease: If the mother is breastfeeding: advise frequent feedings, encourage rooming-in, avoid supplemental water. Do not consider phototherapy in healthy term infants, whether breast-fed or bottle-fed, until bilirubin reaches 25 mg/dL."[5]

Nonetheless, clinicians must remain aware that in rare cases, classic kernicterus has been reported in apparently healthy, full-term, breastfed newborns with no hemolytic disease or other discernible cause for their jaundice.[6]

The current standards used to treat early onset jaundice in the healthy term newborn in the US are based on the AAP Practice Parameter: Management of Hyperbilirubinemia in the Healthy Newborn, published in 1994. This states, "The American Academy of Pediatrics discourages the interruption of breast-feeding in healthy term newborns and encourages continued and frequent breast-feeding (at least eight to ten times every 24 hours). Supplementing nursing with water or dextrose water does not lower the bilirubin level in jaundiced, healthy, breast-feeding infants. Depending on the mother's preference and the physician's judgement, however, a variety of options are presented (below) for possible implementation beyond observation, including supplementation of breast-feeding with formula or the temporary interruption of breast-feeding and substitution with formula, either of which can be accompanied by phototherapy.

AAP Guidelines: Management of hyperbilirubinemia in the healthy term newborn[1] Total serum bilirubin (mg/dL)				
Age, hours	Consider Phototherapy	Phototherapy	Exchange Transfusion	Exchange transfusion and phototherapy
≤24 hours	Clinical jaundice at <24 hours evaluate closely			
25-48	≥12	≥15	≥20	≥25
48-72	≥15	≥18	≥25	≥30
>72	≥17	≥20	≥25	≥30

Hyperbilirubinemia of the term newborn and breastfeeding In addition to complications that can be caused by ineffective breastfeeding, bilirubin levels in the breastfed infant are generally higher than bilirubin levels in the formula-fed infant (0.3% of formula-fed infants will reach a bilirubin of 15.0 mg/dL compared to 2-3% of breast-fed infants).[7,8]   Some experts believe that, as hyperbilirubinemia is universally present in newborns, and physiologic jaundice of the newborn is a normal process, "bilirubin may be an important component of the body's natural defenses against injury by organic free radicals."[9]

The best solution to decrease early onset jaundice is to encourage good hospital policies and practices which support breastfeeding, thus ensuring that the healthy newborn receives adequate breastmilk, and bilirubin levels do not rise to unacceptable levels.

The Baby-Friendly Hospital Initiative, launched by UNICEF and the WHO in 1991, seeks to increase the amount of breastfeeding support in hospitals throughout the world.   The Ten Steps to Successful Breastfeeding (see Appendix) are guidelines hospitals can adopt to ensure maximum breastfeeding promotion and support.

Food for thought

• Normal bilirubin levels vary by ethnicity.   Among blacks and whites, the mean peak of bilirubin levels is 5-6 mg/dL on day three of life.   Among Asians, the mean peak of bilirubin levels is 9-12 mg/dL on day four to five of life.[2]

References

1.   American Academy of Pediatrics.   Practice Parameter: Management of Hyperbilirubinemia in the Healthy Newborn.   *Pediatrics* 1994;94:558-565.

2.   Dixit R, Gardner LM.   The jaundiced newborn: Minimizing the risks. *Contemporary Pediatrics* 1999;16:166-183.

3.   Gartner LM.   Neonatal jaundice.   *Ped in Review* 1994;15:422-432.

4.   Kramer LI.   Advancement of dermal icterus in the jaundiced newborn. *Am J Dis Child* 1969;118:45.

5.   Oski FA.   Hyperbilirubinemia in the term infant: An unjaundiced approach.   *Contemporary Pediatrics* April 1992;148-154.

6.   Auerbach KG.   When treatment for jaundice undermines breastfeeding. *Contemporary Pediatrics* October 1992;105-106.

7.   Maisels MJ, Gifford KL.   Normal serum bilirubin levels in the newborn and the effect of breast-feeding.   *Pediatrics* 1986;78:837.

8.   Maisels MJ, Gifford K, Antle CE, et al.   Jaundice in the healthy newborn infant.   A new approach to an old problem.   *Pediatrics* 1988;81:505.

9.   Schneider AP: Breast milk jaundice in the newborn: a real entity.

JAMA 1986;255:3270.
10. McDonagh AF. Is Bilirubin good for you? *Clinics in Perinatology.* 1990;17:359-369.

Hyperbilirubinemia: late onset ('Breastmilk jaundice')

Summary
Late onset hyperbilirubinemia usually peaks between days seven and 15 of life. When bilirubin levels become unacceptably high, breastfeeding is usually interrupted for 12-24 hours and then resumed.

Definition/cause
'Breastmilk jaundice' refers to late onset hyperbilirubinemia in otherwise healthy breastfeeding infants. Unlike early onset hyperbilirubinemia, which typically peaks around day three of life,[1] breastmilk jaundice begins later and can peak anywhere between days seven and 15 of life, with bilirubin levels usually in the range of 10 to 27 mg/dl.[1]

Although no single causative factor for breastmilk jaundice has been identified, the general perception is that something in the breastmilk triggers the hyperbilirubinemia. Because of an apparent familial tendency, it has been hypothesized that the milk of individual mothers may contain specific causative agents.[1] However, new research suggests that the problem may lie with the infant's genetic makeup rather than with the milk per se. A recent study analyzed the bilirubin uridine diphosphate-glucuronosyltransferase gene (UGT1A1) in infants affected with breastmilk jaundice. A defect in this gene is usually associated with hereditary conditions, such as Gilbert's syndrome, which cause unconjugated hyperbilirubinemia. When researchers analyzed the bilirubin UGT1A1 of 17 otherwise healthy breastfeeding Japanese infants with apparent breastmilk jaundice (total serum bilirubin concentrations above 10 mg/dL) three weeks to one month after birth, they found that 16 of the infants had at least one mutation of the UGT1A1. Researchers concluded that a UGT1A1 defect was an underlying cause of the prolonged unconjugated hyperbilirubinemia associated with breastmilk jaundice, and hypothesized that one or more components in the milk may trigger late onset jaundice in infants who have such mutations.[2]

Another recent study looked at 85 term newborns with unexplained hyperbilirubinemia, who were divided into groups depending on whether they were breast or bottle-fed, and whether they had acute, prolonged, or very prolonged jaundice.   The DNA test for Gilbert's syndrome was performed on all the infants' DNA samples.   The study reported a genetic predisposition to develop prolonged neonatal hyperbilirubinemia in breastfed infants with TATA box polymorphism of the UGT1A1 gene.[3] As a result of these recent findings, many of the questions surrounding breastmilk jaundice may soon be answered.

Signs and symptoms

Typically, infants who develop 'breastmilk jaundice' are thriving, gaining weight, feeding well, and passing abundant stools.   No other clinical abnormalities appear except for high levels of bilirubin.

Treatment

The conventional way to treat breastmilk jaundice is to temporarily halt breastfeeding for 12-24 hours, and to substitute infant formula.[1,4] When breastfeeding is interrupted, bilirubin levels usually fall quickly; when breastfeeding recommences, bilirubin levels will rise somewhat, then slowly begin to decline.

The key question is at what bilirubin level breastfeeding should be interrupted in the otherwise healthy infant, and this decision will depend on the individual clinician's judgement, combined with informed parental opinion.   If the decision is made to interrupt breastfeeding, the mother should be provided with a high quality electric breast pump, and counseled on pumping her milk.   Some sources recommend that the pumped milk be dumped[1] but considering recent findings, there appears to be no reason to believe that milk pumped during this period is any more 'potent' than milk given at any other time.   Logically this milk could be frozen and saved for future use.

Food for thought

• A survey of 886 pediatricians found that physicians with five years or less in practice initiated exchange transfusions at significantly higher serum bilirubin concentrations than physicians who had been practicing for more than five years.[5]

References
1. Lawrence RA, Lawrence RM. *Breastfeeding: A Guide for the Medical Profession.* 5th ed. St. Louis: Mosby; 1999:482-87.
2. Maruo Y, Nishizawa K, Sato H, Sawa H, Shimada M. Prolonged unconjugated hyperbilirubinemia associated with breast milk and mutations of the bilirubin uridine diphosphate-glucuronosyltransferase gene. *Pediatrics* 2000;106(5):E59.
3. Monaghan G, McLellan A, McGeehan A, Li Volti S, Mollica F, Salemi I, et al. Gilbert's syndrome is a contributory factor in prolonged unconjugated hyperbilirubinemia of the newborn. *J Pediatr* 1999;134(4):441-6.
4. Johnson KB, Oski FA. *Oski's Essential Pediatrics.* Philadelphia: Lippincott and Raven, 1997:416-17.
5. Gartner LM, Herrarias CT, Sebring RH. Practice Patterns in Neonatal Hyperbilirubinemia. *Pediatrics* 1998;101(1):25-31.

Infant botulism

Summary
Breastfeeding can continue throughout infant botulism.

Definition/cause
Infant botulism is a rare, acute neurologic disease resulting from a toxin produced by *botulism*, a gram positive, spore forming, obligate anaerobe most commonly found in soil and dust. Infants become infected by inhaling or ingesting the spores. Spore-contaminated honey is an identified source, and infants less than one year of age should not eat honey.

Once ingested, the *Clostridium botulism* spores germinate and multiply in the gut, producing a toxin which is absorbed into the blood stream and blocks acetylcholine release at the neuromuscular junction level, causing paralysis. The toxin irreversibly binds to nerve endings; recovery occurs with the generation of new nerve endings. Seven antigenically distinct toxins have been identified and named A through G. Infant botulism is usually caused by types A and B.

Only 75-100 cases of botulism are diagnosed in the US each year.[1] For unidentified reasons, clinical presentation varies from mild to severe,[2] but most known cases have been serious enough to warrant hospitalization,[2] and in 3% of diagnosed cases, infant botulism is fatal.[1]

The sudden infant death caused by botulism can be confused with the better known sudden infant death syndrome (SIDS or crib death).[2] In California, which has an above average incidence of infant botulism, one out of 20 cases of presumed SIDs cases were found to be due to infant botulism.[3] The age distribution of infant botulism is similar to that of SIDS: 95% of cases occur in infants between three weeks and six months of age, with a peak at between two and four months.[3]

Signs and symptoms

The classic triad seen in infant botulism is constipation, weakness and hypotonicity. Symptoms progress to a symmetric, descending paralysis. To make the diagnosis of infant botulism, the patient must have cranial nerve involvement (termed bulbar palsy).[3] A typical presentation would be an infant less than six months of age who presents with poor feeding and constipation, progressing to difficulty sucking or swallowing (drooling), with an expressionless face, weak cry, loss of gag reflex, poor head control, ptosis and poor tone. The condition is distinguishable from bacterial sepsis in that the patient will be afebrile, with normal mentation.

The diagnosis is made by culturing *Clostridium botulism* from the feces, or testing for the toxin in blood or stool. At the bedside, electromyography (EMG) may be helpful.

Treatment

Once diagnosed, infant botulism is a treatable condition. Botulism immune globulin (BIG), which in the US is available from the Centers for Disease Control,[4] should be administered as soon as possible, to neutralize any unbound toxin. Antibiotics are not used because altering gut flora may increase the amount of toxin in the gastrointestinal tract and worsen the disease.[1]

Infant botulism is a self-limiting illness, usually lasting from two to six weeks, during which time the severely ill patient will need aggressive respiratory and nutritional therapy.[1]

Breastfeeding and infant botulism

Infants diagnosed with botulism can breastfeed or receive pumped breastmilk.[5]

A possible association between breastfeeding and botulism has long been discussed. However, it is unclear whether breastfeeding increases the incidence of infant botulism,[6] or, as current theories suggest, protects against it.[2,7]

Case reports primarily involve infants who are brought to the hospital suffering from botulism,[3] or infants who die a SIDs-like death and are found to have been suffering from undiagnosed botulism.

Arnon,[2] an expert on botulism, reviewed 137 cases of infant botulism resulting from type A or B botulinal toxin, and found that 52% of infants admitted to the hospital were breastfeeding at least five times a day at the onset of illness. Of patients hospitalized in California, the majority of the study group, 66%, were still being nursed at onset of illness. The rate of breastfeeding in matched control infants was significantly fewer: in other words, infants hospitalized with botulism were being breastfed at a higher rate than infants from the general population who were not hospitalized with botulism.[2] It is from such associations that breastfeeding has been suspected of contributing to the frequency of botulism. However, in the same study, none of the ten infants who suffered sudden infant deathlinked to botulism had received human milk for at least ten weeks before death, and eight of them had never been breastfed. All ten were being fed iron-supplemented formula at the time of death, and were formula feeding at a higher rate than matched controls.[2]

Other interesting points included the fact that breastfed infants were twice as old as formula fed infants at the mean age of onset of the disease, and their symptoms were milder.[2] The author suggests, "human milk (or possibly other factors associated with breastfeeding) may have moderated the severity at onset of infant botulism, allowing time for hospital admission, where as for some infants formula milk (or possibly other factors associated with formula feeding) may have permitted sudden onset and unexpected death."[2]

In vitro, the growth of *Clostridium botulinum* is inhibited by *Bifidobacterium* species; also, *Clostridium botulinum* and its toxin production decrease with lowered pH. Human milk encourages the growth of *Bifidobacterium* species, while formula stools have few *Bifidobacterium* species. Human milk stools also have a lower pH (5.1-5.4) than formula based stools (5.9 - 8.0).[5]

Food for thought

The *Clostridium botulinum* toxin is "most potent poison known," 10 pg causes death in mice and 100 ng causes disease in humans. The toxin is killed by heat and pressure (100 degrees C for 10 minutes or 80 degrees C for 30 minutes).[1]

- Between 1977 and 1985, California led the US with the most reported cases of infant botulism (631); Pennsylvania was second (153). However, the states with the highest incidence of infant botulism (cases per 100,000 live births per year) were Delaware (11.0), Hawaii (10.3), Utah (8.3), California (7.1) and Pennsylvania (5.2).[3]

References

1. McMillan JA, DeAngelis DC, Feigin RD, Warshaw JB, eds. *Oski's Pediatrics: Principles and Practice.* 3rd ed. Philadelphia: Lippincott Williams and Wilkins; 1999:940:42.
2. Arnon SS, Damus K, Thompson B, Midura TF, Chin J. Protective role of human milk against sudden death from infant botulism. *J Pediatr* 1982;100(4):568-73.
3. Feigin RD, Cherry, JD eds. *Textbook of Pediatric Infectious Diseases.* 4th ed. Philadelphia: Saunders, 1998:1571-77.
4. American Academy of Pediatrics. In: Pickering LK, ed. *2000 Red Book: Report of the Committee on Infectious Diseases.* 25th ed. Elk Grove Village, IL:American Academy of Pediatrics; 2000:212-214.
5. Lawrence RA, Lawrence RM. *Breastfeeding: A Guide for the Medical Profession.* 5th ed. St. Louis: Mosby, 1999:567.
6. Golding J, Emmett PM, Rogers IS. Does breast feeding protect against non-gastric infections? *Early Hum Dev* 1997;49 Suppl:S105-20.
7. Hanson LA. Human milk and host defence: immediate and long-term effects. *Acta Paediatr Suppl* 1999;88(430):42-6.

Influenza ('Flu)

Summary

A mother with influenza can breastfeed.

Definition/cause

Influenza is an acute respiratory illness caused by the influenza virus.   Three strains of the virus exist, termed A, B, or C.   'Flu epidemics are usually due to the A and B strains; the A virus is associated with the most severe disease, and has been responsible for the worst 'flu epidemics in history.
Influenza is most commonly transmitted through airborne droplets spread by coughing and sneezing, or by poor hygiene.   At the peak of the illness, there are 1,000,000 virus particles per milliliter in respiratory secretions.[1]   Outbreaks tend to occur annually in the winter months, and the most frequent and serious complication is viral or bacterial pneumonia, which can be lethal in high-risk populations. Other complications include otitis media and sinusitis.[1]

Signs and symptoms

Influenza has an abrupt onset: patients can often remember exactly when they started to feel sick.   The illness usually lasts about one week, and symptoms include fever, chills, cough, headache, sore throat, nasal congestion, myalgia, and malaise.

Treatment

Symptomatic treatment consists of rest, fluids, and anti-pyretics as directed by the clinician.   The antiviral medications amantadine and rimantadine can be used as preventive therapy against influenza A, and appear to reduce the duration of the illness if taken within 48 hours of the onset of symptoms.   No side effects of either medication have been reported in breastfeeding infants, although there are no studies of their use in breastfeeding infants.[2]

An inactivated influenza vaccination, made from the influenza A and B viruses present in the previous 'flu season, is available annually in many nations to be given in the fall.   It is recommended for high risk individuals older than six months, including diabetics, patients with chronic cardiovascular and pulmonary disorders, and anyone over 65 years of age.   According to Hale, "There are no reported side effects, nor published contraindications for using influenza virus vaccine during lactation."[2]   More recently, two new neuraminidase inhibitors, zanamivir and oseltamivir have been introduced to shorten the duration, and reduce the severity of influenza infections.   No data are available on levels in human milk.   Further, these agents only lessen the duration of infection by one or two days at best, and their use in otherwise healthy breastfeeding mothers is not necessarily recommended.[2]

Influenza and breastfeeding

By the time the breastfeeding mother realizes she has the 'flu, a highly infectious phase – the 24 hours immediately preceding the onset of symptoms - has already passed.   She will continue to be infectious for several days; the viral shedding in nasal secretions ends approximately seven days after the onset of illness.[3] Breastfeeding protects against upper and lower respiratory tract infections,[4-12] and the antibodies the mother makes against her illness will protect the infant through her milk.   Breastfeeding should continue; however, the mother will need to rest, and to keep herself well hydrated: taking the baby into bed and getting extra help around the house would both help.   Although the mother can take some measures to minimize infection, such as good handwashing, and not coughing or sneezing directly onto the infant, the child is at high risk of infection.

Parents should watch the infant for signs of illness: in infants the flu can present as a minor cold or as a significant infection with high fever.   Parents should contact the doctor when concerned, and particularly if hydration becomes difficult, if the fever becomes hard to control, or if the infant's condition does not begin to improve as the illness progresses.   The infant with 'flu should continue to breastfeed.

Food for thought
• In 1918-1919, influenza A caused one of the worst 'flu epidemics on record.   The outbreak resulted in more than 20 million deaths worldwide, with 550,000 deaths in the USA..[1]
• Children with the 'flu sometimes complain of calf tenderness and refuse to walk (acute myositis).[3]

References
1.   Feigin RD, Cherry, JD eds. *Textbook of Pediatric Infectious Diseases.* 4th ed. Philadelphia: Saunders, 1998:2024-41.
2.   Hale TW.   *Medications and Mothers' Milk.*   9th ed. Amarillo: Pharmasoft Publishing, 2000.
3.   American Academy of Pediatrics.   In: Pickering LK, ed. *2000 Red Book: Report of the Committee on Infectious Diseases.* 25th ed. Elk Grove Village, IL:American Academy of Pediatrics; 2000:351-59 .

4. Forman MR, Graubard BI, Hoffman HJ, Beren R, Harley EE, Bennett P. The Pima infant feeding study: breastfeeding and respiratory infections during the first year of life. *Int J Epidemiol* 1984;13(4):447-53.
5. Burr ML, Limb ES, Maguire MJ, Amarah L, Eldridge BA, Layzell JC, et al. Infant feeding, wheezing, and allergy: a prospective study. *Arch Dis Child* 1993;68(6):724-8.
6. Ford K, Labbok M. Breast-feeding and child health in the United States. *J Biosoc Sci* 1993;25(2):187-94.
7. Golding J, Emmett PM, Rogers IS. Does breast feeding protect against non-gastric infections? *Early Hum Dev* 1997;49 Suppl:S105-20.
8. Hanson LA. Human milk and host defence: immediate and long-term effects. *Acta Paediatr Suppl* 1999;88(430):42-6.
9. Howie PW, Forsyth JS, Ogston SA, Clark A, Florey CD. Protective effect of breast feeding against infection. *BMJ* 1990;300(6716):11-6.
10. Victora CG, Smith PG, Vaughan JP, Nobre LC, Lombardi C, Teixeira AM, et al. Evidence for protection by breast-feeding against infant deaths from infectious diseases in Brazil. *Lancet* 1987;2(8554):319-22.
11. Victora CG, Smith PG, Barros FC, Vaughan JP, Fuchs SC. Risk factors for deaths due to respiratory infections among Brazilian infants. *Int J Epidemiol* 1989;18(4):918-25.
12. Victora CG, Kirkwood BR, Ashworth A, Black RE, Rogers S, Sazawal S, et al. Potential interventions for the prevention of childhood pneumonia in developing countries: improving nutrition. *Am J Clin Nutr* 1999;70(3):309-20.

Inverted nipples

Summary

Women with inverted nipples should be encouraged to breastfeed, but may need extra support from a lactation specialist.

Definition/cause

Nipples come in a variety of shapes and sizes.   Most stick out from the breast; inverted nipples do not: with differing degrees of severity, they are anchored in place by internal adhesions or fibrous tissues, which prevent them from everting.

'True' inverted nipples have been defined as those which retract into the breast when pressure is put onto the areola.[1,2]   The incidence of 'inverted or non-protractile nipples' is commonly cited as being 10%.[3] However, this figure originates from an obscure PhD thesis.[4] A more recent study found congenital inverted nipples in 3.3% of 1625 women. In 87% of these cases, the condition was bilateral.[5]

Much of the research on inverted nipples has been done in the field of plastic surgery. One study reviewed 107 cases of visibly inverted nipples in 60 women, and divided the type of inversion into three categories. 'Grade 1' nipples were easily pulled out manually, and maintained their projection. Most inverted nipples fell into 'grade 2': they could be pulled out but could not maintain projection and tended to recede. Least common were 'grade 3' type nipples, which were difficult to pull out manually because of severe fibrosis beneath the nipple.[6]

Inverted nipples are often established prenatally or in early infancy;[7] in other cases nipple inversion occurs during puberty or adulthood.[8] Some cases of recent inversion in adulthood have been linked with cancer. Sometimes inverted nipples are associated with varied genetic syndromes.[9,10]

Signs and symptoms

Some nipples are so tightly inverted that they turn back into the breast and are barely visible. Other nipples look flat or inverted but will become erect when stimulated, or when the infant starts to suck.

The 'pinch test' can be used to check for a 'true' inverted nipple. To perform the pinch test, the clinician places the thumb below the nipple and the first finger above the nipple, about 2 cm away from the nipple. When gentle pressure is applied by both digits, the inverted nipple will retract into the breast.

In addition to the 'true inverted nipple', some women have a deep groove, almost a 'slit' across the nipple, which has a tendency to become painfully abraded when compressed by the infant's mouth.

Treatment
Prenatal interventions

According to current data, the best prenatal treatment for inverted nipples is to leave them alone.[3,11] In the past, two interventions were widely recommended.

Hoffman's exercises, first used in the 1950s, entail "placing the thumb, or the forefingers, close to the inverted nipple, then pushing into the breast tissue quite firmly and gradually pushing the fingers away from the areola."[12] Hoffman recommended that the exercise be repeated regularly, five times in the horizontal and five times in the vertical plane, with the aim of breaking down the adhesions that keep the nipple inverted.

Breast shells are shallow, dome-shaped cups which fit over the breast and under the bra, with a hole at the center for the nipple (See Breastfeeding aids). The recommendation is that they be worn for short periods of time, to put pressure on the areola at the base of the nipple. In theory this pressure breaks down internal adhesions and everts the nipple.

A randomized controlled trial found that neither Hoffman's exercises nor breast shells were any more effective at everting the nipple than simply leaving it alone.[3] The same study found that treating inverted nipples prenatally with breast shells actually had a *negative* effect on breastfeeding success. More shell-wearers decided prenatally to formula-feed, and only 29% of shell-wearers were breastfeeding six weeks after delivery, compared to 50% of women who did not use shells.[3] The authors concluded that recommending nipple preparation with breast shells may reduce the chances of successful breastfeeding.

Another study of 463 pregnant women in the UK and Canada found no difference in breastfeeding rates at six weeks postpartum between women who left the nipples alone, used Hoffman's exercises, or wore breast shells during pregnancy. The authors concluded, "there is no basis for recommending the use of either Hoffman's nipple stretching exercises or breast shells as antenatal preparation for women with inverted and nonprotractile nipples who wish to breast feed."[11]

Surgery

Inverted nipples can be surgically corrected, but most surgical techniques focus on appearance,[13-17] rather than on maintaining breastfeeding function.[18-20] The degree of inversion can influence the type of surgery used, and whether or not the ducts are cut.[6] Little is known about the breastfeeding rates of women who have surgery to correct an inverted nipple, although some women have successfully nursed after the surgical procedure, even when ducts were severed.[21]

Postpartum guidance and interventions

Rather than attempting to physically correct an inverted nipple prenatally, the clinician can best help the mother by offering accurate anticipatory guidance to prepare her for the best possible chance of breastfeeding success. The mother should try to put the infant to breast immediately after birth: unless the inversion is severe, the baby may be able to latch and nurse. Once the newborn successfully latches onto a flat or inverted nipple, the mother would be well advised to avoid artificial nipples – bottles and pacifiers – especially in the early days, to prevent the infant from becoming accustomed to a long, hard, artificial teat.

If one nipple protrudes and the other is inverted, the mother can breastfeed primarily on the side that functions effectively, while continuing to offer the inverted nipple on a regular basis. If the baby is extremely hungry, it makes sense to offer the easier option. If the baby is calm and looking more for comfort than for nourishment, the inverted side might be tried. A baby can be nourished on one breast; indeed some cultures breastfeed exclusively on one breast.[22] However, as the baby grows and the nursing dyad becomes more experienced, the baby may eventually pull out and nurse successfully on the inverted nipple.

Minor postpartum interventions include manual stimulation or ice on the areola or nipple to create an erect nipple. An inverted syringe with one end cut off can be placed with the smooth side over the nipple; as the piston is gently pulled out the nipple will evert, possibly far enough to allow the infant to latch (see Breastfeeding aids). For the 'grooved' nipple, experimentation may reveal a position in which the infant can suck on the nipple without compressing it and causing abrasion. If the nipple is already sore, Lansinoh™ cream (purified lanolin recommended for sore nipples) can be used in the short term to cover raw skin and ease the pain.

Where the inversion is severe and latching continues to be unsuccessful, a good quality electric breast pump (see Breastfeeding aids) is the best long term solution. The pump will help to pull out the nipple, and will stimulate the breast to begin producing milk. If the baby cannot latch at all despite intensive lactation support, the mother can pump and collect milk to feed the infant by an alternative method.

Inverted nipples and breastfeeding

Although flat nipples are sometimes difficult for the infant to grasp, a well-latched infant who has taken a large amount of the areola into the mouth can often pull out a flat or slightly receding nipple and nurse well.   However, if the nipple retreats out of reach when the infant compresses the areola, breastfeeding can be difficult. The mother should be referred to experienced lactation support, and the infant's weight carefully monitored after discharge.   In cases of severe inversion, full breastfeeding may not be possible and continued supplementation, either with the mother's own pumped milk, or with formula if the mother is unable to produce enough milk, may be necessary.[2]

Prior to going home, the mother with inverted nipples should be thoroughly counseled on signs of adequate hydration in her child. She should be advised to look for at least three stools and six to eight wet diapers in 24 hours (once the infant is greater than 72 hours old). Early follow-up is warranted, and the mother should know where to call if she has concerns. Nipple stimulation sends messages to the brain which results in the release of prolactin and oxytocin. If the nipple is inverted, it receives less stimulation which may lead to decreased milk supply.   Inverted nipples have been associated with dehydration in breastfeeding newborns. In one in-depth review of five exclusively breastfed infants re-admitted to hospital with severe dehydration and hypernatremia, three of the mothers had inverted nipples, and all three experienced difficulties with proper latch early postpartum.   One of the three infants had lost 32% of birthweight when dehydration was diagnosed at 14 days of life, and had not been seen by a pediatrician for a weight check, although the mother had called the pediatrician's office with breastfeeding questions.   The infant developed multiple cerebral infarctions and had decreased facial movements on follow up.   The other two babies lost 26% and 16% of birth weight at days nine and five of life respectively, and neither had been seen by a pediatrician since initially going home from the hospital.[23]

Food for thought

• A nipple splint is a device used in plastic surgery to maintain postoperative appearance of corrected inverted nipples.[13]

References

1. Lawrence RA, Lawrence RM. *Breastfeeding: A Guide for the Medical Profession.* 5th ed. St. Louis: Mosby; 1999:247-48.
2. Riordan J, Auerbach KG. *Breastfeeding and Human Lactation.* 2nd ed. Sudbury: Jones and Bartlett; 1999:98.
3. Alexander JM, Grant AM, Campbell MJ. Randomized controlled trial of breast shells and Hoffman's exercises for inverted and non-protractile nipples. *BMJ* 1992;304(6833):1030-2.
4. Alexander JM. The prevalence and management of inverted and non-protractile nipples in antenatal women who intend to breastfeed. PhD theseis. University of Southampton, 1991.
5. Park HS, Yoon CH, Kim HJ. The prevalence of congenital inverted nipple. *Aesthetic Plast Surg* 1999;23(2):144-6.
6. Han S, Hong YG. The inverted nipple: its grading and surgical correction. *Plast Reconstr Surg* 1999;104(2):389-95; discussion 396-7.
7. James T. Curiosa paediatrica V: Inverted nipples. *S Afr Med J* 1981;60(15):598.
8. Kalbhen CL, Kezdi-Rogus PC, Dowling MP, Flisak ME. Mammography in the evaluation of nipple inversion. *AJR Am J Roentgenol* 1998;170(1):117-21.
9. Lorenzetti MH, Fryns JP. Inverted nipples in Robinow syndrome. *Genet Couns* 1996;7(1):67-9.
10. Fryns JP, Aftimos S. New MR/MCA syndrome with distinct facial appearance and general habitus, broad and webbed neck, hypoplastic inverted nipples, epilepsy, and pachygyria of the frontal lobes. *J Med Genet* 2000;37(6):460-2.
11. Preparing for breast feeding: treatment of inverted and non-protractile nipples in pregnancy. The MAIN Trial Collaborative Group. *Midwifery* 1994;10(4):200-14.
12. Hoffman JB. A suggested treatment for inverted nipples. *Am J Obstet Gynec* 1953;66:346-8.
13. De Lorenzi C, Halls MJ. A nipple splint. *Plast Reconstr Surg* 1988;81(6):959-60.
14. Rayner CR. The correction of permanently inverted nipples. *Br J Plast Surg* 1980;33(4):413-7.
15. Pribaz JJ, Pousti T. Correction of recurrent nipple inversion with cartilage graft. *Ann Plast Surg* 1998;40(1):14-7.
16. Aiache A. Surgical repair of the inverted nipple. *Ann Plast Surg* 1990;25(6):457-60.
17. Pompei S, Tedesco M. A new surgical technique for the correction of the inverted nipple. *Aesthetic Plast Surg* 1999;23(5):371-4.
18. el Sharkawy AG. A method for correction of congenitally inverted nipple with preservation of the ducts. *Plast Reconstr Surg*

1995;95(6):1111-4.
19. Kami T, Wong AC, Kim IG. A simple method for the treatment of the inverted nipple. *Ann Plast Surg* 1988;21(4):316-21.
20. Sakai S, Sakai Y, Izawa H. A new surgical procedure for the very severe inverted nipple. *Aesthetic Plast Surg* 1999;23(2):139-43.
21. Terrill PJ, Stapleton MJ. The inverted nipple: to cut the ducts or not? *Br J Plast Surg* 1991;44(5):372-7.
22. Ing R, Petrakis NL, Ho JH. Unilateral breast-feeding and breast cancer. *Lancet* 1977;2(8029):124-7.
23. Cooper WO, Atherton HD, Kahana M, Kotagal UR. Increased incidence of severe breastfeeding malnutrition and hypernatremia in a metropolitan area. *Pediatrics* 1995;96(5 Pt 1):957-60.

Low milk supply

Summary

Breastfeeding can continue if the mother's milk supply is low, but the infant will probably need supplementation.   Measures should be taken to increase the milk supply.

Definition/cause

A mother whose milk supply is inadequate is not producing enough milk to meet her baby's needs.   Many causes exist for low milk supply; the most common is mismanagement of breastfeeding.[1]   Breastfeeding mismanagement can result from offering fewer than eight feeds in 24 hours, limiting the amount of time spent at the breast, rigidly scheduling feeds, poor latch, formula supplementation, overuse of pacifiers, and from hospital routines which do not support breastfeeding.

Other maternal conditions which can result in low supply include a history of breast surgery, retained placental fragments, certain medications (such as ergot alkaloids), use of estrogen-containing birth control pills, inverted nipples (see Inverted nipples), Sheehan's syndrome (see Sheehan's syndrome), and, rarely, lactation failure due to breast hypoplasia or other factors.

Inadequate milk supply can also occur in women who are pumping, either long term for a premature or otherwise hospitalized infant, or at work.   A poor quality breast pump, or infrequent use of a breast pump can both cause insufficient breast stimulation, which will in turn lead to a reduction in milk supply.

Signs and symptoms

Symptoms of low milk supply in the new mother are difficult to evaluate. On the first day postpartum, a woman produces about 50 mL (three tablespoons) of colostrum, and her breasts show little sign of fullness. On day two, she produces about 250 mL of colostrum. Many women interpret this normal situation as inadequate supply.[2] Even later during lactation, attempts at hand expression, or use of a breast pump, are both unlikely to produce more than a few mL of milk on the mother's first attempts. A mother may hand express inefficiently, and she often needs time to become used to a pump, thus measuring milk supply with these methods is unlikely to be accurate. It is easier to spot signs of insufficient milk supply in the mother by watching the infant.

In the newborn period, insufficient milk intake is indicated by weight loss greater than 7%,[3] fewer than two stools per 24 hours, and other signs of dehydration (see Dehydration). A newborn who is not receiving enough milk will have inadequate weight gain and may fail to regain birth weight by two weeks of age.

In the early weeks of life, underfed infants gain weight poorly and usually demonstrate one of two opposing behaviors. Some infants, often enthusiastically but erroneously described as 'good babies' by their parents, are constantly sleepy, regularly napping for long periods between feeds, and eating fewer than eight times per day. Other infants fuss constantly, rarely sleep for more than half an hour at a time, cry frequently, nurse continually, and never appear satisfied.

Later during lactation, if a mother's milk supply dips after a return to work, for example, a baby may show signs of frustration at the breast, nursing only for a brief period, then pulling off the breast and crying. The mother is usually reliable when reporting a decreased output if she is pumping regularly for the older baby, because she witnesses less pumped milk.

Signs of the rarer but pathological lactation failure include lack of breast changes during pregnancy (such as increase in size, darkening of the areola, and increased visibility of blood vessels); marked absence of engorgement, and undeveloped or unequal breasts.

Treatment
Inadequate intake in the newborn.

Prior to discharge, the new breastfeeding mother needs to hear consistent, accurate anticipatory guidance from hospital staff.   She should breastfeed her baby at least eight to twelve times in 24 hours, and by day four to five of life, she should see at least three stools and six or more wet diapers in 24 hours.   In addition, a follow up appointment and weight check should be made for the newborn 48-72 hours after discharge.[4]

Before discharge, the infant's weight should be monitored.   All neonates lose weight.   However, if the weight loss is greater than 7%,[3] questions should be raised about intake.   Not all newborns need immediate supplementation at this point.   Sometimes the breastfeeding gets off to a poor start.   For example, a mother may have a difficult recovery from a cesarean birth, but after the first couple of days, her child may start to nurse well.   The experienced clinician may feel comfortable sending this infant home without supplementation but with an early appointment for a weight check.   However, if a mother is having trouble with positioning or latch, the child's weight is continuing to dip below 7%, and the breastfeeding is clearly not going well, supplementation with formula may be needed.   The decision to supplement with formula at this point is not without controversy. Frequent nursing, extra stimulation, for example with a breast pump, and referral to an experienced lactation consultant in the community are all options that can be considered.   However, in the authors' experience of working in an inner city hospital with a low income, high risk population, such options are not always available to all mothers.

Similarly, if an infant is seen soon after going home, is continuing to lose weight, and is not on track to regain birth weight by two weeks of life, the child will probably need supplementation, initially at least, with the mother's pumped milk, with banked human milk where it can be obtained, or with infant formula.

A hungry, underweight baby can be offered the breast first at each feed, but should subsequently receive as much supplement as s/he will take, as often as s/he will take it.

Raising the milk supply: fixing mismanagement

The best remedy for low milk supply due to breastfeeding

mismanagement is to increase the number of feeds at breast: in other words, to offer the breast more frequently. Pacifiers, which encourage non-nutritive sucking, should be eliminated. In addition, use of a good quality electric breast pump bilaterally for ten minutes after each feed will stimulate breastmilk production. Any milk pumped can be given as a supplement. If the parents wish to avoid bottles, supplements of either pumped milk or formula can be offered after a breastfeed, by cup or syringe. They can also be offered using the Supplemental Nursing System ™ (see Breastfeeding aids). If the infant can latch and suck, the SNS™ is a good option because the infant is still receiving all nourishment at breast, and stimulating the breast. In most cases, the mother's milk supply rebounds with the additional stimulation, and supplements can gradually be discontinued.

If the mother's milk supply does not rebound with a combination of extra feeding and pumping, maternal factors (see **Definition/cause**) should be more thoroughly examined.

Pumping mothers and inadequate supply

Diminished supply among women relying on a breast pump can often be remedied by increasing the number of pumpings, and by ensuring that the mother is using a top quality pump. Among mothers of infants hospitalized in the NICU, kangaroo care or skin-to-skin holding – where the premature or sick infant is placed between the mother's breasts, wearing only a diaper, then covered for warmth – has been shown to boost milk supply.[5,6]

Medications and galactogogues

Certain medications can also improve supply: metoclopramide (Reglan), frequently used to treat gastroesophageal reflux, appears to stimulate basal prolactin levels, which leads to increased milk production at a dose of 30-45 mg per day.[7,8] In one study of 32 women, metoclopramide augmented milk supply in approximately 67% of mothers who reported lactation failure (no milk, or only drops of milk, after nursing for at least one week) and in 100% of women with insufficient milk.[9] In another study of 23 mothers with hospitalized premature infants and faltering milk supply, metoclopramide effectively increased milk production in 100% of cases.[10]

Metoclopramide should be prescribed by a physician with full knowledge of the mother's medical history, such as her primary care doctor or her obstetrician.   The recommended dose is 30-45 mg per day, which could be started as 10-15 mg three times per day.[8] Usually, metoclopramide is recommended for a maximum of four weeks because of the increased possibility of side effects, which can include maternal depression, stomach cramping, and diarrhea.[8]   If the medication is stopped abruptly, milk production may decline significantly, so tapering the dose over one to two weeks is recommended.[8]   No side effects have been reported in the infants of mothers using metoclopramide, which is commonly prescribed for babies and children.[8]

Given the recommendation for short term administration, metoclopramide is useful as a 'booster' for diminished milk supply, in combination with increased frequency of breastfeeding when possible.

The authors have had success using this drug among mothers pumping long term for infants in the NICU; among exclusively pumping mothers whose milk supply was never successfully established, and, in one case, with a mother who lost custody of her infant for six weeks, during which time she pumped to maintain a milk supply.   The psychological boost provided by a visible increase in milk supply encouraged these women to augment the rigorous pumping regime necessary to ensure a more permanent return of the milk supply.

Another known galactogogue is the medication domperidone,[11-14] which is available in many countries (though not in the USA) and is often considered safer than metoclopramide because it does not cross the blood brain barrier.[13] Like metoclopramide, domperidone is a peripheral dopamine antagonist, which is known to increase prolactin levels and to increase milk supply.[12-14] The suggested dose in order to increase milk supply is 20-40 mg orally, three to four times per day.[8]

The herb fenugreek (*trigonella foenum graecum*) is also a touted galactogogue.   Sold as a dried seed, taken as a tea, and used as a cooking spice, fenugreek is frequently reported by lactation consultants to increase milk supply.   The one study to date on fenugreek's galactagogue properties found that three capsules of fenugreek seed, taken three times daily for one week by ten women, increased average daily milk volume (measured against milk volume in the same women when not taking fenugreek) from 207 mL to 464 mL.[15]   Possible side effects in the adult include diarrhea, hypoglycemia, and dyspnea. Fenugreek has a maple syrup flavor, and can cause a maple syrup odor in sweat and urine in mother and infant, which can lead to confusion with maple syrup urine disease.[16] No side effects have thus far been recorded in infants of mothers using fenugreek.[8]

Low milk supply and breastfeeding

Ensuring appropriate prenatal education, educating health care professionals to provide accurate, consistent breastfeeding advice, eliminating formula discharge packs, and creating hospital routines that support breastfeeding could eliminate many of the breastfeeding mismanagement problems which lead to low milk supply.[17-25] In the NICU setting appropriate guidance is particularly important, and programs are needed to increase support for mothers who choose to provide breastmilk for their high-risk infants.[26-29]

Food for thought

- The number one reason mothers quit breastfeeding in the hospital following birth is an erroneously *perceived* lack of milk supply.[2]
- Fenugreek has been shown to reduce postprandial glucose levels in non-insulin dependent diabetics,[30] and significantly reduced fasting blood sugar and improved the glucose tolerance test in insulin dependent diabetics.[31]
- Popular but unproven galactogogues in varied cultures include: beer or brewer's yeast (USA), anise and cotton seeds (Mexico), seaweed soup (Korea), and goat's stomach (Pakistan).[32]

References

1. Powers NG. Slow weight gain and low milk supply in the breastfeeding dyad. Clin Perinatol 1999;26(2):399-430.
2. Winikoff B, Myers D, Laukaran VH, Stone R. Overcoming obstacles to breast-feeding in a large municipal hospital: Applications of lessons learned. Pediatrics 1987;80(3):423-33.
3. DeMarzo S, Seacat I, Neifert M.   Initial weight loss and return to birth-weight criteria for breast-fed infants: Challenging the "rules of thumb". Am J Dis Child 1991;145(402).
4. American Academy of Pediatrics, Work Group on Breastfeeding. Breastfeeding   and   the   Use   of   Human   Milk.   Pediatrics

1997;100(6):1035-1039.
5. Anderson GC. Current knowledge about skin-to-skin (kangaroo) care for preterm infants. J Perinatol 1991;11(3):216-26.
6. Charpak N, Ruiz-Pelaez JG, Figueroa de Calume Z. Current knowledge of Kangaroo Mother Intervention. Curr Opin Pediatr 1996;8(2):108-12.
7. Kauppila A, Kivinen S, Ylikorkala O. A dose response relation between improved lactation and metoclopramide. Lancet 1981;1(8231):1175-7.
8. Hale TW. Medications and Mothers' Milk. 9th ed. Amarillo: Pharmasoft Publishing, 2000.
9. Gupta AP, Gupta PK. Metoclopramide as a lactogogue. Clin Pediatr (Phila) 1985;24(5):269-72.
9. Ehrenkranz RA, Ackerman BA. Metoclopramide effect on faltering milk production by mothers of premature infants. Pediatrics 1986;78(4):614-20.
11. Brown TE, Fernandes PA, Grant LJ, Hutsul JA, McCoshen JA. Effect of parity on pituitary prolactin response to metoclopramide and domperidone: implications for the enhancement of lactation. J Soc Gynecol Investig 2000;7(1):65-9.
12. Petraglia F, De Leo V, Sardelli S, Pieroni ML, D'Antona N, Genazzani AR. Domperidone in defective and insufficient lactation. Eur J Obstet Gynecol Reprod Biol 1985;19(5):281-7.
13. Hofmeyr GJ, Van Iddekinge B, Blott JA. Domperidone: secretion in breast milk and effect on puerperal prolactin levels. Br J Obstet Gynaecol 1985;92(2):141-4.
14. Hofmeyr GJ, van Iddekinge B. Domperidone and lactation. Lancet 1983;1(8325):647.
15. Effect of fenugreek on breast milk volume. Academy of Breastfeeding Medicine Fifth Annual Meeting; 2000 September 11-13; Tuscon, Arizona.
16. Sewell AC, Mosandl A, Bohles H. False diagnosis of maple syrup urine disease owing to ingestion of herbal tea. N Engl J Med 1999;341(10):769.
17. Philipp BL, Merewood A, O'Brien S. US physicians and the promotion of breastfeeding: A Call for Action. Pediatrics In press.
18. Howard CR, Schaffer SJ, Lawrence RA. Attitudes, practices, and recommendations by obstetricians about infant feeding. Birth 1997;24(4):240-6.
19. Howard FM, Howard CR, Weitzman M. The physician as advertiser: the unintentional discouragement of breast-feeding. Obstet Gynecol 1993;81(6):1048-51.
20. Freed GL, Clark SJ, Cefalo RC, Sorenson JR. Breast-feeding education of obstetrics-gynecology residents and practitioners. Am J Obstet Gynecol 1995;173(5):1607-13.
21. Freed GL, Clark SJ, Lohr JA, Sorenson JR. Pediatrician involvement in

breast-feeding promotion: a national study of residents and practitioners. Pediatrics 1995;96(3 Pt 1):490-4.

22. Cooper WO, Atherton HD, Kahana M, Kotagal UR. Increased incidence of severe breastfeeding malnutrition and hypernatremia in a metropolitan area. Pediatrics 1995;96(5 Pt 1):957-60.

23. Bick DE, MacArthur C, Lancashire RJ. What influences the uptake and early cessation of breast feeding? Midwifery 1998;14(4):242-7.

24. Merewood A, Philipp BL.   Implementing change: becoming Baby-Friendly in an inner city hospital. Birth 2001;28(1).

25. Frank DA, Wirtz SJ, Sorenson JR, Heeren T. Commercial discharge packs and breast-feeding counseling: effects on infant-feeding practices in a randomized trial. Pediatrics 1987;80(6):845-54.

26. Schanler RJ, Hurst NM, Lau C.   The use of human milk and breastfeeding in premature infants. Clin Perinatol 1999;26(2):379-98, vii.

27. Lawrence PB. Breast milk. Best source of nutrition for term and preterm infants. Pediatr Clin North Am 1994;41(5):925-41.

28. Meier PP, Brown LP. State of the science. Breastfeeding for mothers and low birth weight infants. Nurs Clin North Am 1996;31(2):351-65.

29. Philipp BL, Brown E, Merewood A. Pumps for Peanuts: Leveling the Field in the NICU. Jnl of Perinatology 2000;4:249-250.

30. Madar Z, Abel R, Samish S, Arad J.   Glucose-lowering effect of fenugreek in non-insulin dependent diabetics.   Eur J Clin Nutr 1988;42(1):51-4.

31. Sharma RD, Raghuram TC, Rao NS. Effect of fenugreek seeds on blood glucose and serum lipids in type I diabetes.   Eur J Clin Nutr 1990;44(4):301-6.

32. Riordan J, Auerbach KG. Breastfeeding and Human Lactation. 2nd ed. Sudbury: Jones and Bartlett, 1999:41-42.

Mastitis

Summary

Breastfeeding can continue unrestricted throughout episodes of mastitis. The mother should be evaluated by a clinician.

Definition/cause

Sporadic puerperal mastitis is an acute cellulitis, characterized by a fever, and caused in approximately half of cases by *Staphylococcus aureus*,[1,2] or less frequently by *Streptococcus*. Development is

150

strongly associated with sore or cracked nipples.[3,4] An association also exists between mastitis and milk stasis, which can result from unresolved engorgement or plugged ducts.[2,5,6] Fatigue, stress, and restrictive clothing which put pressure on the breast are commonly cited as causes of mastitis, but these associations have not been closely studied.

Discrepancy exists in the medical literature around the incidence of mastitis, with some studies finding rates in approximately 3% of the breastfeeding population,[1,7] and others citing an incidence of 20-25%.[3,8,9] This discrepancy may be due in part to differing criteria concerning the definition of mastitis. For example, not all affected women reported fever in Vogel's study,[8] yet fever is usually included in the definition of mastitis.

Signs and symptoms

Symptoms include a fever, often over 101° F; a painful, inflamed quadrant, usually on one breast, which is generally inflamed and warm to the touch; and general achiness or flu-like signs in the mother. Mastitis differs from plugged ducts in that it involves fever and systemic malaise in addition to localized pain.

Treatment

Treatment consists primarily of antibiotic therapy,[10] which will clear the infection and prevent abscess formation.[1,2] Because the most common organism in infectious mastitis is staphylococcal in origin, antibiotics such as nafcillin, dicloxacillin, cloxacillin, and flucloxacillin, with specific coverage of staphylococcal infections, are recommended. None of these medications would be expected to cause problems for infants of breastfeeding mothers.[11] In addition, the mother should breastfeed frequently to drain the affected breast, rest, drink plenty of fluids, and use comfort measures such as pain medication and warm compresses.

Mastitis and breastfeeding

Breastfeeding should continue throughout episodes of mastitis: interrupting breastfeeding can cause engorgement, which may contribute to abscess formation.

Resolving mastitis involves more than prescribing antibiotics: the clinician should discuss prevention and potential causes of mastitis with the mother – for example, unresolved plugged ducts, or missed feedings, and assist her in finding ways to reduce risk factors for repeated episodes.

References
1. Marshall BR, Hepper JK, Zirbel CC. Sporadic puerperal mastitis. An infection that need not interrupt lactation. *JAMA* 1975;233(13):1377-9.
2. Niebyl JR, Spence MR, Parmley TH. Sporadic (nonepidemic) puerperal mastitis. *J Reprod Med* 1978;20(2):97-100.
3. Jonsson S, Pulkkinen MO. Mastitis today: incidence, prevention and treatment. *Ann Chir Gynaecol Suppl* 1994;208:84-7.
4. Livingstone V, Stringer LJ. The treatment of Staphyloccocus aureus infected sore nipples: a randomized comparative study. *J Hum Lact* 1999;15(3):241-6.
5. Lawrence RA, Lawrence RM. *Breastfeeding: A Guide for the Medical Profession.* 5th ed. St. Louis: Mosby, 1999:277-82.
6. Riordan J, Auerbach KG. *Breastfeeding and Human Lactation.* 2nd ed. Sudbury: Jones and Bartlett, 1999:485-87.
7. Kaufmann R, Foxman B. Mastitis among lactating women: occurrence and risk factors. *Soc Sci Med* 1991;33(6):701-5.
8. Vogel A, Hutchison BL, Mitchell EA. Mastitis in the first year postpartum. *Birth* 1999;26(4):218-25.
9. Kinlay JR, O'Connell DL, Kinlay S. Incidence of mastitis in breastfeeding women during the six months after delivery: a prospective cohort study. *Med J Aust* 1998;169(6):310-2.
10. Thomsen AC, Espersen T, Maigaard S. Course and treatment of milk stasis, noninfectious inflammation of the breast, and infectious mastitis in nursing women. *Am J Obstet Gynecol* 1984;149(5):492-5.
11. Hale TW. *Medications and Mothers' Milk.* 9th ed. Amarillo: Pharmasoft Publishing, 2000.

Multiples

Summary
Mothers of twins and sometimes of triplets can usually produce enough milk to feed their infants, but practical support is invaluable.

Definition/cause
All types of multiple births have increased dramatically in the US

over the past three decades.   Between 1971 and 1997, twins births increased by 53% in whites, 32% in African Americans, 31% in Native Americans, and 83% in Mexican American women.   Triplet, quadruplet, and quintuplet (or higher order) births increased by 400%, 1100%, and 500%, respectively.[1] The increase in multiple births can be ascribed to successful fertility treatments, particularly in vitro fertilization (IVF),[2] and to the increasing age of the maternal cohort.[1]

The increase in multiple births has created a corresponding increase in preterm and low birth weight infants, and has impacted US infant mortality figures.[1,2]   Nine out of 10 triplets are born preterm compared with one in 10 singletons. The average triplet weighs 1,698 grams at birth, half that of the average singleton (3,358 grams), and triplets are about 12 times more likely to die during the first year of life.[3]

Multiples and breastfeeding

Mothers of multiples must deal with two major challenges: milk levels and energy levels.   Twin mothers and some triplet mothers are usually physically capable of producing enough milk for their infants.[4,5]   The problem is rarely production, it is more likely to be exhaustion, especially bearing in mind that many multiple births are premature or problematic, involving cesarean births or smaller than average newborns who may be sleepy or developmentally incapable of suckling efficiently from birth.

These mothers will need generous emotional support, as well as practical tips on breastfeeding two or more babies.   The clutch or football hold allows the mother to nurse two babies simultaneously, with one tucked under each arm.   A nursing pillow that fits around the waist and provides basic support may aid some mothers. Although adding a breast pump to the picture may seem overwhelming, it can be useful.   If the infants are born prematurely, the breastfeeding mother will need a pump (see Prematurity).   In addition, a high quality breast pump can help to stimulate the maternal milk supply in the early days if the babies are not latching well, and can provide milk for supplements if these become necessary for small or sleepy infants.

Parents of multiples may want to keep a log of feedings and of stools, which will remind and reassure them of each child's nursing sessions and output.

Offering realistic anticipatory guidance to parents who are expecting twins is paramount. The elderly primagravida who has used fertility treatments may idealize the newborn period: however, the reality is less straightforward. Research shows that at four months postpartum, women who conceived by IVF reported lower self-esteem, lower maternal self-efficacy, and considered their infants as more temperamentally difficult than women who conceived without fertility treatment.[6] Before the birth, parents can contact multiple birth support groups, and arrange for help at home, particularly in the newborn period. Support in the hospital is also worth considering. A helpful partner, friend or grandparent is invaluable if, for example, the woman who has a cesarean birth is rooming in with her twins. It is unrealistic to expect such a mother to be able to cope alone.

Food for thought

- Between 1971 and 1994 the number and ratio of triplet births quadrupled, rising from 1,034 to 4,594, and from 29.1 to 116.2 per 100,000 live births.[3]
- Massachusetts reported the highest triplet birth ratio with 215.9 per 100,000 live births, more than twice the U.S. ratio.[3]
- Author Dr. Bobbi Philipp gave birth to twins (a girl and a boy) weighing almost 8 lb each. She says, "It is possible to breastfeed twins!" Her advice: "Get help, and enjoy!"

Resources

Mothering multiples: Breastfeeding and Caring for Twins or More! *By Karen Gromada. La Leche League International, US $14.95.*

Parenting multiples online:
http://multiples.miningco.com/parenting/multiples/mbody.htm

Mothers of Supertwins (MOST)
P.O. Box 951
Brentwood, NY 11717-0627
631/859-1110
www.mostonline.org/index.htm

The Triplet Connection
PO Box 99571
Stockton CA 95209
209/474-0885
www.webmaster@tripletconnection.org

References
1. Keith LG, Oleszczuk JJ, Keith DM. Multiple gestation: reflections on epidemiology, causes, and consequences. *Int J Fertil Womens Med* 2000;45(3):206-14.
2. Tough SC, Greene CA, Svenson LW, Belik J. Effects of in vitro fertilization on low birth weight, preterm delivery, and multiple birth. *J Pediatr* 2000;136(5):618-22.
3. Martin JA, MacDorman MF, Mathews TJ. Triplet births: trends and outcomes, 1971-94. *Vital Health Stat 21* 1997(55):1-20.
4. Lawrence RA, Lawrence RM. *Breastfeeding: A Guide for the Medical Profession.* 5th ed. St. Louis: Mosby; 1999:469-70.
5. Riordan J, Auerbach KG. *Breastfeeding and Human Lactation.* 2nd ed. Sudbury: Jones and Bartlett; 1999:326-28.
6. McMahon CA, Ungerer JA, Tennant C, Saunders D. Psychosocial adjustment and the quality of the mother-child relationship at four months postpartum after conception by in vitro fertilization. *Fertil Steril* 1997;68(3):492-500.

Neural tube defect (Myelodysplasia)

Summary
An infant with a neural tube defect can breastfeed. If the infant is physically unable to breastfeed, the infant can receive expressed breastmilk.

Definition/cause
The fetal nervous system begins developing on the 18th day of gestation and neural tube closure is normally is completed by 23-28 days of gestation. A failure of neural tube closure during this time produces defects of varying severity in differing anatomical locations.

The cause of neural tube defects is unknown, but there appears to be a genetic predisposition; after one child in a family is born with a meningomyelocele, the risk of recurrence is 3-4%; after two affected pregnancies, the risk rises to 10%.[1]

Until recently, neural tube defects were among the most common congenital malformations affecting newborns.   However, over the past 30 years the incidence has fallen significantly.   For example, in England and Wales in 1970, 4.5 neural tube defects occurred per 1,000 live births; by 1991, the rate had fallen to 0.18 per 1,000 live births.[2] This decrease is due to a combination of prenatal diagnosis and elective termination of affected pregnancies, and to periconceptional folate therapy: maternal supplementation with folic acid greatly reduces the incidence of neural tube defects.[2]

Neural tube defects are more prevalent among certain ethnic groups including Sikhs, Hispanics, those with Irish ancestry, and Northern American and Alaskan natives.[3]

Characteristics

Anencephaly.   In this lethal neural tube defect, the brain never forms correctly.   The bones of the cranial vault are absent, and cerebral and cerebellar hemispheres, brainstem, and basal ganglia are absent or only rudimentary.   An infant born with this condition will not develop and usually dies shortly after birth.

Encephalocele.   In this condition, the infant is born with a gap in the skull and herniation of brain.   Most infants with encephalocele do not survive long, or are severely mentally retarded, however, early surgery can sometimes create a better prognosis.

Spina bifida is the most common neural tube defect.   It usually presents as a herniation (a 'ballooning out of soft tissue') of either the meninges (a 'meningocele'), the spinal cord (a 'myelocele'), or of both the meninges and the spinal cord (myelomeningocele or meningomyelocele) through the gap in the spine.   This last is the most common presentation of spina bifida, occurring in approximately 80% of affected babies, and affecting 0.2 to 0.4 per 1000 live births.[2] In 69% of cases the abnormality is located in the lumbar and lumbosacral area, and 75% of the time it is associated with hydrocephalus.[2] Paralysis of the lower limbs results from damage to the spinal cord, and depending on the site of the lesion, the condition may be associated with secondary orthopedic malformations of the lower extremities, which occur in utero due to the lack of fetal movement.   Other possible complications include abnormalities of brain structure, abnormal bladder innervation, precocious puberty, growth hormone deficiency, bowel incontinence, and chronic constipation.

Spina bifida occulta. In this presentation there is no protrusion of the spinal cord or its membrane, although a hairy tuft, dimple or unusual pigmentation may be visible on the infant's back. This condition is often associated with a delay in walking, abnormal anatomy of the leg or foot, and back or leg pain.[2]

Treatment

A newborn with spina bifida will usually have surgery to close the spinal defect within 24 hours of birth, in order to minimize the risk of infection and to preserve existing spinal cord function. Other surgeries and extensive medical care may be necessary throughout life. Children with spina bifida will need to learn mobility skills through the use of crutches, braces, or wheelchairs. Because some degree of neurological damage may be present, as the child grows, psychological evaluation will be useful, as will early interventional strategies.

Neural tube defects may be diagnosed in utero or at birth. Alpha fetoprotein (AFP) produced by the fetus leaks into the amniotic fluid through the neural tube defect and then diffuses into the maternal circulation. If maternal serum AFP screening tests, drawn between the 15th and 18th week of gestation, reveal elevated AFP levels, an ultrasound or an amniotic AFP is obtained to confirm a possible neural tube defect.[1]

Prevention is the best measure for countering neural tube defects. Folic acid (folate) is involved in the conversion of homocysteine to methionine; elevated levels of homocysteine have been shown to be associated with neural tube defects. Consumption of folic acid for at least three months before conception and during the first month of pregnancy has been shown to reduce the occurrence of neural tube defects by 50-72%.[4,5] The U.S. Public Health Service currently recommends that all women of childbearing age consume 400 micrograms (0.4 mg) of folic acid daily. Folic acid is available in dark leafy green vegetables, and is added to some foods, such as enriched breads, pastas, rice, and cereals.[6]

Neural tube defects and breastfeeding

Even when an infant is terminally ill, the mother may wish to pump breastmilk for her infant. Such wishes should not be overlooked.

For the infant with a better long term prognosis, breastfeeding often proves less challenging than parents may fear from the initial medical diagnosis. The basic reflexes are usually present in infants with spina bifida, and with regard to feeding, these infants often act like any other infant, with effective rooting, sucking and swallowing. The biggest challenges often surround restrictive positioning following early surgery: flexion of the spine may not be possible, and the baby may have to remain flat on the back or on the belly for several days. Lactation consultants experienced with spina bifida suggest that the best post-surgical solution is for the mother to lie beside the infant in the hospital bed, and to feed in the sidelying position, or to slide the child on pillows onto the mother's lap, and from there to devise any kind of breastfeeding position that works to get the nipple into the infant's mouth. (Kimberly Barbas, BSN, IBCLC, Lactation Consultant, Children's Hospital, Boston: personal communication). If necessary, the infant can be tube or bottle fed with pumped breastmilk until post-surgical restrictions are lifted and the baby can be more easily positioned.

As with any infant born with a medical issue, breastfeeding can help to normalize the experience for the mother.

Food for thought
- Latex allergy is common in children with spina bifida.
- Northern Britain has a high incidence of neural tube defects.

Resources
Spina Bifida Association of America
4590 MacArthur Blvd NW, Suite 250
Washington, DC 20007-4226
Tel. 800/621-3141
www.sbaa.org

Latex Allergy Information Service
176 Roosevelt Ave.
Torrington, CT 06790
www.latexallergyhelp.com

www.aplacetoremember.com: Support materials on high risk pregnancy, problems of pregnancy, loss during pregnancy or loss of an infant, and future pregnancies.

www.nationalshareoffice.com: Pregnancy and infant loss support.

References
1. Elias ER, Hobbs N. Spina bifida: Sorting out the complexities of care. *Contemporary Ped* 1998;15:156-171.
2. Taeusch HW, Avery ME. *Avery's Diseases of the Newborn*. 7th ed. Philadelphia:WB Saunders; 2000:399-402.
3. Hall JG, Solehdin F. Folic acid: It's good preventive medicine. *Contemporary Ped* 1998;15:119-136.
4. Czeizel AE, Dudas I. Prevention of the first occurrence of neural tube defects by periconceptual vitamin supplementation. *New Engl J Med* 1992;327:1832.
5. Butterworth CE, Bendich A. Folic acid and the prevention of birth defects. *Annu Rev Nutr* 1996;16:73.
6. CDC:Birth Defects and Pediatric Genetics Branch, National Center for Environmental Health, Centers for Disease Control and Prevention, 4770 Buford Highway, NE, MS F-45, Atlanta, GA 30341-3724. www.cdc.gov/nceh/cddh/folic/default.htm

Nursing strike

Summary
Breastfeeding could continue through a nursing strike, were the baby to oblige.   Since the striking baby does not oblige and refuses to nurse, the mother needs patience and insight to endure and ultimately overcome a nursing strike.

Definition/cause
The so-called nursing strike describes the sudden refusal to breastfeed by a healthy older baby – often aged between seven to nine

months – who has previously been nursing happily. It is often interpreted as weaning, but self-weaning is rare under one year of age, and is usually a gradual process, whereas a nursing strike is sudden. A nursing strike may or may not follow a change in the mother's routine (for example, a return to work); habits (a new perfume or a change in diet); or a biting incident (the baby bites the mother, and the mother reacts with a loud cry) (see Biting and teething).

Before labeling the behavior a nursing strike, medical causes such as a cold (which will cause blocked nostrils and may cause the infant to pull off the breast), thrush, or a painful viral infection such as hand-foot-and-mouth disease should be ruled out.

Signs and symptoms
The previously content older baby suddenly refuses to breastfeed.

Nursing strike and breastfeeding
Little has been published in the medical literature about nursing strikes, but the major breastfeeding texts[1,2] agree on the basic definition and management.

The baby on nursing strike is usually vibrant and healthy, and the refusal to breastfeed is a mystery and a source of distress to the mother. Frequently, babies go on nursing strike at around seven to nine months, an age when nursing sessions usually spell relaxation and enjoyment for the breastfeeding pair. The mother is often understandably distressed when this special time is abruptly forsaken by the baby. With patience and confidence, however, a mother can usually overcome a nursing strike and the baby will return to the breast.[3] Resolution may require several days, and the mother may need to pump meanwhile to relieve engorgement and maintain her milk supply.

Typically nursing strikes follow a predictable pattern. Initially the baby completely refuses to nurse when awake. Treating the baby as a younger infant, with lots of skin to skin care and holding, is the first step towards a return to nursing; once the baby tolerates close holding, s/he can be put to breast whilst sleepy or in light sleep. Within one to two days the sleepy baby will usually begin to accept the breast, and thereafter will begin breastfeeding whilst awake, eventually appearing to forget the incident completely.

Food for thought

- If the mother reports that her four to five month-old infant 'doesn't want to breastfeed', or is constantly pulling off the breast to look around, the baby is probably not 'on strike', but entering a developmental phase of increased curiosity about the world. In time, this phase will pass.
- Infants have been reported to reject the breast and sometimes wean altogether if the mother becomes pregnant again.[4]

References
1. Lawrence RA, Lawrence RM. *Breastfeeding: A Guide for the Medical Profession*. 5th ed. St. Louis: Mosby;1999:343:44.
2. Riordan J, Auerbach KG. *Breastfeeding and Human Lactation*. 2nd ed. Sudbury:Jones and Bartlett;1999:328-29.
3. Winchell K. Nursing strike: misunderstood feelings. *J Hum Lact* 1992;8(4):217-9.
4. Newton N, MT. Breastfeeding during pregnancy in 503 women: does psychobiological weaning mechanism exist in humans? *Emotion Reprod* 1979;20B:845.

Obesity

Summary
Obesity is rarely an issue among healthy, exclusively breastfed infants, and breastfeeding appears to protect against obesity in children.

Definition/cause
Obesity is an excess of body fat, which can be evaluated by calculating weight for height and age.

Treatment
Because obese children often become obese adults, and are likely to carry risk factors for cardiovascular disease,[1] preventative strategies are important. Healthy breastfed infants are almost never obese;[1] if a 'breastfed' infant appears overweight, the parents may be supplementing with either formula or solids,[1] and should be reassured that breastmilk alone can provide adequate nutrition for approximately

the first six months of life.

Obesity and breastfeeding
Preventative effects

Recent research implies that breastfeeding protects against obesity. A study of almost 10,000 German children entering kindergarten found that 4.5% of children who had never been breastfed were obese, compared with 2.8% of breastfed children, and a dose-response effect was identified for the duration of breastfeeding on the prevalence of obesity.[3] Another study reviewed 781 adolescents and found that teenagers who were exclusively breastfed for more than three months were less overweight than adolescents who were breastfed for three months or less.[4]

Women who breastfeed for six months or more lose weight in the postpartum period more quickly than women who do not breastfeed.[5]

Growth patterns and growth charts

Breastfed infants and formula-fed infants grow differently during the first year of life: breastfed infants gain weight more quickly in the first two to three months,[6,7] but are leaner by one year of age.[8] According to the 'DARLING' study, the mean weight of formula-fed infants remained at or above the National Center for Health Statistics median throughout the first 18 months of life, while the mean weight of breastfed infants dropped below the median, beginning at six to eight months, and was significantly lower than that of the formula-fed group between six and 18 months. Length and head circumference were similar in both groups, but the authors noted that according to weight-for-length scores, breastfed infants between four and 18 months were considerably leaner.[9]

The growth charts produced by the National Center for Health statistics in 1977, and used by the vast majority of US pediatricians until 2000, were derived from the Fels Longitudinal Study, and were based on a population of primarily white, formula-fed infants from Ohio. As a result, the growth patterns described were not always accurate for predominantly and exclusively breastfed infants, who would appear to 'fall off' the growth curve at approximately four months of age, when their initially accelerated growth as breastfed infants slowed.

New growth charts from the Centers for Disease Control were produced in 2000, and based on a more heterogeneous population of both breastfed and formula-fed infants; however, few exclusively breastfed children appear to have been included.[10] These new growth charts generally demonstrate higher weights for children between birth and 24 months of life, which, in the words of one commentator, "will accentuate the difference in weight that we already appreciate from the DARLING studies....this might lead to unfortunate consequences. Health care providers might attempt to classify healthy breastfeeding infants as underweight and recommend nutritional supplements and/or weaning to achieve higher weights."[10]

The World Health Organization is currently collecting data from seven international sources, among exclusively or predominantly breastfed infants. Growth charts are expected to be created from this data before 2005.

Maternal obesity

Obese women should be encouraged to breastfeed their infants. Some minor breastfeeding problems have been associated with maternal obesity: one study examined breastfeeding rates in a population of white obese women, and found that among 810 women who ever put their infants to breast, women who were overweight or obese had less success initiating breastfeeding than their normal-weight counterparts. Overweight and obese women also discontinued exclusive breastfeeding earlier, and had a shorter overall breastfeeding duration than women of normal weight. The results remained constant despite controlling for parity, socioeconomic status, and maternal education.[11]

Food for thought

• Approximately 97 million adult Americans are either overweight or obese.

References

1. Freedman DS, Dietz WH, Srinivasan SR, Berenson GS. The relation of overweight to cardiovascular risk factors among children and adolescents: the Bogalusa Heart Study. *Pediatrics* 1999;103(6 Pt 1):1175-82.

2. Lawrence RA, Lawrence RM. *Breastfeeding: A Guide for the Medical Profession.* 5th ed. St. Louis: Mosby, 1999.
3. von Kries R, Koletzko B, Sauerwald T, von Mutius E, Barnert D, Grunert V, et al. Breast feeding and obesity: cross sectional study. *BMJ* 1999;319(7203):147-50.
4. Tulldahl J, Pettersson K, Andersson SW, Hulthen L. Mode of infant feeding and achieved growth in adolescence: early feeding patterns in relation to growth and body composition in adolescence. *Obes Res* 1999;7(5):431-7.
5. Dewey KG, Heinig MJ, Nommsen LA. Maternal weight-loss patterns during prolonged lactation. *Am J Clin Nutr* 1993;58(2):162-6.
6. Dewey KG, Peerson JM, Brown KH, Krebs NF, Michaelsen KF, Persson LA, et al. Growth of breast-fed infants deviates from current reference data: a pooled analysis of US, Canadian, and European data sets. World Health Organization Working Group on Infant Growth. *Pediatrics* 1995;96(3 Pt 1):495-503.
7. Agostoni C, Grandi F, Gianni ML, Silano M, Torcoletti M, Giovannini M, et al. Growth patterns of breast fed and formula fed infants in the first 12 months of life: an Italian study. *Arch Dis Child* 1999;81(5):395-9.
8. Dewey KG, Heinig MJ, Nommsen LA, Peerson JM, Lonnerdal B. Breast-fed infants are leaner than formula-fed infants at 1 y of age: the DARLING study. *Am J Clin Nutr* 1993;57(2):140-5.
9. Dewey KG, Heinig MJ, Nommsen LA, Peerson JM, Lonnerdal B. Growth of breast-fed and formula-fed infants from 0 to 18 months: the DARLING Study. *Pediatrics* 1992;89(6 Pt 1):1035-41.
10. Feldman-Winter L. The new CDC growth charts: how do they measure up for the breastfeeding population? *Academy of Breastfeeding Medicine News and Views* 2000;6(6):17-20.
11. Chapman DJ, Perez-Escamilla R. Identification of risk factors for delayed onset of lactation. *J Am Diet Assoc* 1999;99(4):450-4; quiz 455-6.

Osteogenesis imperfecta (Brittle bone disease)

Summary
An infant with osteogenesis imperfecta (OI) can breastfeed. Lactation support should include assisting the mother with careful positioning.

164

Definition/cause

Osteogenesis imperfecta is an autosomal dominant inherited disorder of connective tissue occurring in 1 out of 20,000 infants. Individuals with this disease produce abnormal type 1 collagen, an important component in bone and skin tissue. Four types of OI exist, with presentation ranging from a severe form associated with death in the perinatal period, to a mild form that may escape diagnosis until adulthood.

Signs and symptoms

The classic triad of symptoms comprises fragile bones, blue sclerae and deafness. The bones break easily, and the newborn may be discharged as healthy after birth, only to return shortly thereafter with severe bruising, lumps, or other symptoms of fractures. X-rays may reveal older fractures caused in utero or during birth.

Complications associated with this disease include easy bruising, joint laxity, recurrent pneumonia, and cardiac failure.

Treatment

Osteogenesis imperfecta cannot be cured; emphasis is on helping the individual lead as full a life as possible.

OI and breastfeeding

Combined with the shock of diagnosis, the parents may experience guilt at having inadvertently broken bones by holding, hugging, and playing with their infant. The mother may be afraid to hold her child and cause further damage. In order to help her during breastfeeding, pillows can be used to create a 'platform', on which the baby can lie while the mother focuses primarily on head control and the finer points of positioning. In a case where family members must limit and control physical contact with the infant, the closeness of breastfeeding assumes a critical nurturing role. Kangaroo care, where the infant lies prone, skin to skin on the parent's chest, should be discussed with the parents as a safe and calming way to increase physical contact with their fragile infant.

Food for thought
• Until the correct diagnosis is made, child abuse may be suspected because of the multiple fractures associated with OI .

Resources
Osteogenesis Imperfecta Foundation
804 West Diamond Ave., Ste. 210
Gaithersburg, MD 20878
800/981-2663
301/947-0083
www.oif.org

References
1. Behrman RE, Kliegman RM, Jenson, HB eds. *Nelson Textbook of Pediatrics*, 16th ed. Philadelphia:WB Saunders 2000:2128-30.

Phenylketonuria (PKU)

Summary
An infant with PKU should be fed a phenylalanine-free formula, supplemented by partial breastfeeding as determined by regular monitoring of serum phenylalanine levels.

Definition/cause
Phenylketonuria (PKU) is an autosomal recessive disorder found in approximately 1:10,000 children in the United States. Those with Northern European ancestry have an increased incidence; for example, the incidence is 1:6,000 in Ireland and Scotland. Newborn screening for PKU is performed in many countries, including all US states, the District of Columbia, Puerto Rico and the US Virgin Islands. To be accurate, screening should be performed when the infant is more than 24 hours of age.[1]

PKU was first reported in 1934 by Norwegian physician and biochemist, Asbjorn Folling, and is known as Folling's disease in Norway.[2] Infants with PKU lack the liver enzyme phenylalanine hydroxylase (PAH), and cannot convert phenylalanine to tyrosine in protein metabolism. These two amino acids are the precursors of important compounds like thyroid hormone, neurotransmitters, and melanin.   When PAH is missing or defective, phenylalanine or its abnormal breakdown products like phenylacetic acid and phenylpyruvic acid (phenylketones) build up in the blood and urine. Phenylketones are harmful to the cells of the developing nervous system.   Phenylalanine is an essential amino acid; some is necessary for normal function but it cannot be synthesized in the body.

Signs and symptoms

If untreated, the disease causes developmental delay in the first year of life, progressing to severe mental retardation (95% of untreated patients have an IQ below 50).   Untreated PKU will also cause seizures, autistic-like behavior, eczema-like rashes, uneven pigmentation, a peculiar musty blood and urine odor, and a reduced life span.

Treatment

Normal development occurs if the patient follows a diet low in phenylalanine.   Dietary intervention should begin before the infant is four weeks of age (optimally, as soon as possible), and treatment centers on adapting the infant's diet so it contains enough phenylalanine for essential needs but no more than the body can handle.[3,4,5]

PKU and breastfeeding

Breastmilk contains less phenylalanine than formula, but it contains too much to be the exclusive nutritional source.   Ideally, the mother should offer a phenylalanine-free formula, supplemented with as much breastmilk as allowed.   The balance of phenylalanine-free formula versus breastmilk is determined by regularly monitoring the infant's serum phenylalanine levels and adjusting intake accordingly. In most cases, individuals with PKU are followed by a physician who specializes in this disorder.

Newborns who received only breastmilk *prior to diagnosis and treatment for PKU* were shown to have 12.9 more IQ points when adjusted for social and maternal education status.[6,7]

Food for thought

- Pearl Buck, Nobel and Pulitzer Prize author of *The Good Earth*, wrote about the mysterious illness that affected her daughter, Carol, in another of her books, *The Child Who Never Grew*. Carol was eventually diagnosed with PKU around 1960, when screening tests were administered at her residence, the New Jersey Vineland Training School for the Mentally Retarded.(2)
- Folling discovered that the urine of a child with PKU, loaded with phenylketones, would turn blue-green when ferric chloride was added.
- The artificial sweetener, aspartame (NutraSweet), is contraindicated in a PKU diet.

Resources

Children's PKU Network
1520 State St., Ste. 111
San Diego, CA 92101
Tel. 619/233-3202

References

1. American Academy of Pediatrics, Committee on Genetics. Newborn Screening Fact Sheets. *Pediatrics* 1996;98:473-501.
2. Centerwall SA, Centerwall WR. The discovery of phenylketonuria: The story of young couple, two retarded children and a scientist. *Pediatrics* 2000;105:89-103.
3. Clark BJ. After a positive Guthrie – what next? Dietary management for the child with phenylketonuria. *Eur J Clin Nutr* 1992;46 (supp 1):533-539.
4. Ernest AE, McCabe ERB, Neifert MR, et al. Guide to Breastfeeding the Infant with PKU. (DHHS Publication No. 79-5110) Washington, US Government Printing Office, 1980.
5. Duncan LL, Elder SB. Breastfeeding the infant with PKU. *J Hum Lact* 1997;13(3):231-5.
6. Riva E, Agostoni C, Biasucci G, et al. Early breastfeeding is linked to higher intelligence quotient scores in dietary treated phenylketonuric children. *Acta Paediatr* 1996;85:56-8.
7. Agostoni C. Early breastfeeding linked to higher intelligence quotient scores. *Acta Paediatr* 1996;85:639.

Pierre Robin syndrome

Summary

The mother of an infant with Pierre Robin syndrome should be encouraged to provide breastmilk for her baby. However, the combination of cleft palate and glossoptosis makes successful breastfeeding unlikely.

Definition/cause

Pierre Robin syndrome is a congenital condition involving a triad of micrognathia (an abnormally small mandible), glossoptosis (irregular tongue position), and a high arched or cleft palate. Its alternative nomenclature, Pierre Robin sequence, refers to the theory that the abnormal formation of the mandible, which happens seven to 11 weeks after conception, leads to secondary malformation of the palate and tongue in the fetus.[1] Many affected infants have other irregularities including congenital glaucoma, and heart anomalies. Thirty percent of affected individuals have Sticklers syndrome, an autosomal dominant disorder associated with early arthritis and eye problems.[2]

The severity of the syndrome varies tremendously from patient to patient. While some infants die perinatally, others can be managed with only minor intervention.[3]

Characteristics

The infant with Pierre Robin syndrome has a small, receded mandible, which self corrects in childhood, but the angle of the jaw remains abnormal throughout life. Infants with this syndrome usually have airway issues and breathing difficulties,[4] especially if in a supine position, due to posterior rotation of the tongue,[5] which falls backwards and blocks the airway. Chronic airway obstruction can lead to failure to thrive, or to severe respiratory distress.[4] Twenty percent of affected individuals suffer from mental retardation, although some of these incidences may be due to early asphyxia.[2] Other complications include gastroesophageal reflux[5] and chronic ear infections: patients should be monitored closely for middle ear disease leading to potential hearing loss and delayed speech.[1]

One study divided 125 children identified with Pierre Robin syndrome into three groups depending on the severity of their symptoms. Some 44.8% were able to breathe and feed orally (though all were reported as 'bottle feeding') when placed in the prone position; 32% were able to breathe well when prone but required gavage feeding, and 23.2% required endotracheal intubation and gavage feedings. Of the 125 cases, 13% died, most of them from the group with the most severe symptoms, and half had at least one other anomaly besides the Pierre Robin triad.[3]

Treatment

Infants with this syndrome require careful airway and feeding management, as well as eventual surgical repair of the cleft palate when present.

Feeding problems in infants may need to be resolved by gavage tube, or by aids such as the Haberman™ feeder, which does not require suction to deliver milk into the mouth (see Breastfeeding aids). Breathing difficulties may be resolved by surgical placement of a tracheostomy (see Tracheostomy), or by a procedure known as glossopexy, in which the tongue is attached to the lower lip and mandible to prevent it from blocking the upper airway. Glossopexy is performed early in infancy and reversed at the time of palatal repair, usually at around one year of age.[6] Less invasive management includes possible placement of a nasogastric tube for airway maintenance and supplementation of oral feeding.[7]

Infants who do not require a tracheostomy may need to be kept and fed in a prone position for several months until the mandible grows and relieves the glossoptosis.

Pierre Robin syndrome and breastfeeding

The possibility of successful breastfeeding in infants with this and closely related syndromes depends on the severity of the symptoms, but in most cases, successful breastfeeding is unlikely.[8]

Many of these babies do not feed orally at all and require gavage tubes. Infants who can eat by mouth are hampered by the combination of a cleft palate, which makes it difficult to form a seal (see Cleft lip and cleft palate), and the abnormal tongue which makes 'milking' the breast difficult. Some children are able to feed orally using a special device such as a Haberman™ feeder, or by using a bottle with an enlarged hole.[9] The authors were unable to locate any published reports of successful breastfeeding in infants with Pierre Robin syndrome. As long as nutrition is guaranteed and the infant is placed in a safe position to allow for glossoptosis, however, there is no reason to discourage the mother from attempting to breastfeed.

Whether or not the infant is able to suckle, the clinician should encourage the mother to obtain a high quality electric breast pump (see Breastfeeding aids), and begin to pump her breasts to provide breastmilk for the baby. If the baby is unable to nurse, the mother will need to double pump approximately every three hours for 10-15 minutes in order to create and maintain a milk supply. The mother should be informed that human milk will help to protect the susceptible infant from infections, especially those associated with abnormal crano-facial development.

Food for thought

- The triad of micrognathia, cleft palate, and respiratory obstruction was first described in 1822.[1]
- In 1923, French stomatologist Pierre Robin coined the term glossoptosis to describe the classic way in which the tongue fell backwards and blocked the airway in infants with this syndrome.[1]
- Pierre Robin syndrome is one of more than 300 differing 'cleft syndromes'.[2]

Resources

Children's Craniofacial Assoc.
PO Box 280297
Dallas, TX 75228
800/535-3643
972/994-9902
www.masterlink.com\children

Craniofacial Foundation of America
C/O Terri Farmer
975 E. Third St.
Chattanooga TN 37403
800/418-3223
423/778-9192
www.erlanger org/cranio

FACES-The National Craniofacial Assoc.
PO Box 11082
Chattanooga TN 37401
800/332-2372
412/266-1632
www.faces-cranio.org

Let's Face It
PO Box 29972
Bellingham, WA 98228
360/676-7325
www.faceit.org/faceit/

National Foundation for Facial Reconstruction
317 E. 34th St., Rm. 901
New York, NY 10016
212/263-6656
www.nffr.org

References

1. Taeusch HW, Avery ME. *Avery's Diseases of the Newborn.* 7th ed. Philadelphia:WB Saunders, 2000: 43-45.
2. Syndromes with oral manifestation in Nelson Textbook of Pediatrics. 16th edition. Philadelphia:WB Saunders:2000:1113.
3. Caouette-Laberge L, Bayet B, Larocque Y. The Pierre Robin sequence: review of 125 cases and evolution of treatment modalities. *Plast Reconstr Surg* 1994;93(5):934-42.
4. Bath AP, Bull PD. Management of upper airway obstruction in Pierre Robin sequence. *J Laryngol Otol* 1997;111(12):1155-7.
5. Dudkiewicz Z, Sekula E, Nielepiec-Jalosinska A. Gastroesophageal reflux in Pierre Robin sequence--early surgical treatment. *Cleft Palate Craniofac J* 2000;37(2):205-8.
6. LeBlanc SM, Golding-Kushner KJ. Effect of glossopexy on speech sound production in Robin sequence. *Cleft Palate Craniofac J* 1992;29(3):239-45.
7. Prodoehl DC, Shattuck KE. Nasogastric intubation for nutrition and airway protection in infants with Robin sequence. *J Perinatol* 1995;15(5):395-7.
8. Lawrence RA, Lawrence RM. *Breastfeeding: A Guide for the Medical Profession.* 5th ed. St Louis:Mosby;1999:491.
9. Singer L, Sidoti EJ. Pediatric management of Robin sequence. *Cleft Palate Craniofac J* 1992;29(3):220-3.

Plugged ducts

Summary

Breastfeeding should be encouraged throughout episodes of plugged ducts. The mother should be watched for signs of mastitis.

Definition/cause

A 'plugged duct' occurs when a milk duct inside the breast becomes blocked, and milk collects behind the plug. No one specific cause of plugged ducts has been identified; frequently quoted associations among lactation professionals with clinical experience include fatigue, engorgement, nursing in an awkward position, and chronic external pressure on the breast (for example, from a baby carrier or a tight bra).

Signs and symptoms

A plugged milk duct causes a painful, sometimes red and swollen lump, in a localized area of one breast, which usually resolves within 24 – 48 hours of appropriate therapy. Unresolved plugged ducts can lead to mastitis;[1] clinicians should warn the patient to watch for the systemic signs which distinguish mastitis from a plugged duct: fever over 101 degrees; aching, flu-like symptoms, localized warmth, and increasing discomfort in the breast (see Mastitis).

Treatment

Treatments for plugged ducts include increasing the amount of nursing on the affected side, manually massaging the site, applying warm compresses, and soaking the affected breast in warm water. Nursing first on the affected side, in order to take advantage of the infant's strongest sucking, is sometimes advised.

Plugged ducts and breastfeeding

Plugged ducts are, for the most part, temporary annoyances for the breastfeeding mother. Chronic plugged ducts should be investigated as to cause. The prime concern is that plugged ducts may develop into mastitis.

Food for thought

- Some experts recommend pointing the baby's nose towards the plug while breastfeeding for maximum sucking strength.[1]
- When the plug unblocks, the milk may leave the breast in long, spaghetti-like strands.

References

1. Riordan J, Auerbach KG. *Breastfeeding and Human Lactation.* 2nd ed. Sudbury: Jones and Bartlett; 1999:484-86.

Postpartum depression

Summary

Breastfeeding can continue in women with postpartum depression. However, the mother needs treatment and support, and her breastfeeding status should be considered when medications are prescribed.

Definition/cause

'Postpartum depression' has been categorized into three separate states: postpartum 'blues', postpartum depression, and postpartum psychosis.[1] Problems arise when true postpartum depressive disorders are dismissed as normal physiologic changes associated with childbirth, and women fail to receive appropriate treatment.[1]

Many women suffer some degree of 'baby blues' after childbirth, but studies disagree on exactly how many women experience these feelings: reported rates vary from 30-84%.[2] The 'blues' usually appear around the third day postpartum, are temporary, have only a minor functional impact, and respond well to social support.[1,3] By contrast, postpartum depression, which usually peaks later,[4] can significantly compromise daily function and does not easily resolve without professional support. Studies estimate that 7-14% of women develop postpartum depression.[4,5] The most extreme disorder, postpartum psychosis, occurs when patients develop psychosis, mania, or thoughts of infanticide.[1]

Several factors predict the possibility of postpartum depression. A past history of psychiatric or depressive disorders is one significant risk factor;[6-8] other predictors can include a family history of depression, social adjustment, and stressful life events.[7] Generally, the postpartum period is a high-risk time for recurrence of depression, mania, or psychosis for women with bipolar disorder.[9]

Hormonal influences are believed to play a role in postpartum depression.[8,10] 'The blues' are commonly blamed on dramatic postnatal hormonal fluctuations. One study found that women with postpartum depression had significantly lower plasma prolactin levels than those without depression, and women who developed depression six to ten weeks after giving birth had significantly lower plasma prolactin and significantly greater progesterone levels than those who were not depressed.[8]

Signs and symptoms

The postpartum 'blues' are usually temporary, occur at around three days postpartum, and can involve fluctuating moods, strong emotions, and weepiness.[1]

Postpartum depression generally peaks at around ten weeks postpartum,[4] and symptoms include anxiety, despair, insomnia, feelings of inadequacy, hopelessness and helplessness, reduced appetite, irrationality, and suicidal thoughts.[2,3]

Postpartum psychosis occurs when women develop psychosis, mania, or thoughts of infanticide;[1] they may also have delirium, confusion, hallucinations, and threaten suicide.[2,3] The onset of psychosis is generally between two and eight weeks postpartum.[2]

Postpartum depression in the mother has been associated with adverse emotional and cognitive development in the infant.[2]

Treatment

Women whose personal history contains risk factors for postpartum depression require careful follow-up. If postpartum depression (beyond the 'blues') develops, medication and psychotherapy are usually warranted. Puerperal prophylaxis with mood stabilizers or antidepressants in the early postpartum period is thought to decrease the risk of recurrent depression, mania, or psychosis for women with bipolar disorder.[9,11]

Antidepressant medications and breastfeeding

A thorough review of psychiatric medications and breastfeeding can be found in Hale's *Clinical Therapy in Breastfeeding Patients.*[12]

A review of all papers published between 1993 and 1998 on the use of psychotropes in breastfeeding women found both tricyclic antidepressants (TCA) and specific serotonin re-uptake inhibitors (SSRIs) relatively safe in breastfeeding women.[11] However, high-dose antipsychotics were thought to be associated with long-term adverse sequelae in the infant.[11]

Of the SSRIs, sertraline (Zoloft) appears to be the safest for nursing mothers.[12] Fluoxetine (Prozac) has a long half-life of 24-36 hours, and it is largely metabolized to norfluoxetine, which has a half life of approximately 360 hours. Fluoxetine and norfluoxetine both permeate breastmilk with milk/plasma ratios varying from 0.28 to as high as 0.67. Several reports of colic, tremulousness, insomnia, and other severe side effects have been reported following the use of fluoxetine in newborns.[13,14] By contrast, although sertraline has a half-life of 26-65 hours, its metabolite, desmethylsertraline, is only marginally active, and levels of sertraline and desmethylsertraline in the milk appear to be low, with a milk/plasma ratio of around 0.89.[12,15]

Other SSRIs generally considered safe for breastfeeding women include paroxetine, venlafaxine, and citalopram, although several reported cases of somnolence have been reported for citalopram.[12] Clomipramine, which is used for panic disorders and obsessive-compulsive disorders, is approved by the American Academy of Pediatrics for use in breastfeeding women.

Postpartum depression and breastfeeding

The woman with postpartum depression can continue to breastfeed, but will need professional support. Postpartum depression has been associated with compromises in the mother-infant relationship;[16-18] in addition, significant associations between maternal depression and lower rates of infant cognitive development have been recorded. Maternal depressive symptoms at seven weeks postpartum predicted lower infant social and performance scores at three months. Maternal moods at six months were associated with lower scores in infant motor development at the same age.[19] Several studies have found an association between postpartum depression and shortened breastfeeding duration.[20-23] In a study of 159 mothers, longer breastfeeding duration was significantly associated with lower levels of anxiety and depression, and increased self-esteem and coping capacity.[21]   Another study found that while depression was not linked with the decision to breastfeed, it was associated with early cessation of breastfeeding.[22]

Tamminen found that depressed mothers reported more breastfeeding problems than other women.[5] Looking at the same issue from a different perspective, a study of 258 English women who initiated breastfeeding found that those who were still breastfeeding at three months postpartum were less likely to suffer from depression or fatigue than women who had weaned.[24]

Food for thought

- A review of 12 trials found that a doula (a trained birth assistant) positively influenced the mother's psychological state in the postpartum period.   Eight of the studies reported early or late psychosocial benefits of the doula, including decreased symptoms of depression, reduced anxiety, increased breastfeeding initiation, and increased maternal sensitivity to the child's needs.[25]
- The Edinburgh Postnatal Depression Scale is a short questionnaire developed to help clinicians distinguish between postpartum depression and the more common, less serious baby 'blues'.

References

1. Susman JL. Postpartum depressive disorders. *J Fam Pract* 1996;43(6 Suppl):S17-24.
2. Lawrence RA, Lawrence RM. *Breastfeeding: A Guide for the Medical Profession*. 5th ed. St. Louis: Mosby; 1999:551-56.
3. Riordan J, Auerbach KG. *Breastfeeding and Human Lactation*. 2nd ed. Sudbury: Jones and Bartlett, 1999:564-68.
4. Pop VJ, Essed GG, de Geus CA, van Son MM, Komproe IH. Prevalence of post partum depression--or is it post-puerperium depression? *Acta Obstet Gynecol Scand* 1993;72(5):354-8.
5. Tamminen T.   The impact of mother's depression on her nursing experiences and attitudes during breastfeeding. *Acta Paediatr Scand Suppl* 1988;344:87-94.
6. O'Neill T, Murphy P, Greene VT. Postnatal depression--aetiological factors. *Ir Med J* 1990;83(1):17-8.

7. O'Hara MW, Schlechte JA, Lewis DA, Wright EJ. Prospective study of postpartum blues. Biologic and psychosocial factors. *Arch Gen Psychiatry* 1991;48(9):801-6.
8. Abou-Saleh MT, Ghubash R, Karim L, Krymski M, Bhai I. Hormonal aspects of postpartum depression. *Psychoneuroendocrinology* 1998;23(5):465-75.
9. Chaudron LH, Jefferson JW. Mood stabilizers during breastfeeding: a review. *J Clin Psychiatry* 2000;61(2):79-90.
10. Susman VL, Katz JL. Weaning and depression: another postpartum complication. *Am J Psychiatry* 1988;145(4):498-501.
11. Austin MP, Mitchell PB. Use of psychotropic medications in breast-feeding women: acute and prophylactic treatment. *Aust N Z J Psychiatry* 1998;32(6):778-84.
12. Hale TW. *Clinical Therapy in Breastfeeding Patients.* Amarillo: Pharmasoft Publishing, 1999.
13. Taddio A, Ito S, Koren G. Excretion of fluoxetine and its metabolite, norfluoxetine, in human breast milk. *J Clin Pharmacol* 1996;36(1):42-7.
14. Lester BM, Cucca J, Andreozzi L, Flanagan P, Oh W. Possible association between fluoxetine hydrochloride and colic in an infant. *J Am Acad Child Adolesc Psychiatry* 1993;32(6):1253-5.
15. Hale TW. *Medications and Mothers' Milk.* 9th ed. Amarillo: Pharmasoft Publishing, 2000.
16. Nagata M, Nagai Y, Sobajima H, Ando T, Nishide Y, Honjo S. Maternity blues and attachment to children in mothers of full-term normal infants. *Acta Psychiatr Scand* 2000;101(3):209-17.
17. Cooper PJ, Tomlinson M, Swartz L, Woolgar M, Murray L, Molteno C. Post-partum depression and the mother-infant relationship in a South African peri-urban settlement. *Br J Psychiatry* 1999;175:554-8.
18. Sugawara M, Kitamura T, Toda MA, Shima S. Longitudinal relationship between maternal depression and infant temperament in a Japanese population. *J Clin Psychol* 1999;55(7):869-80.
19. Galler JR, Harrison RH, Ramsey F, Forde V, Butler SC. Maternal depressive symptoms affect infant cognitive development in Barbados. *J Child Psychol Psychiatry* 2000;41(6):747-57.
20. Murray L, Sinclair D, Cooper P, Ducournau P, Turner P, Stein A. The socioemotional development of 5-year-old children of postnatally depressed mothers. *J Child Psychol Psychiatry* 1999;40(8):1259-71.
21. Galler JR, Harrison RH, Biggs MA, Ramsey F, Forde V. Maternal moods predict breastfeeding in Barbados. *J Dev Behav Pediatr* 1999;20(2):80-7.
22. Papinczak TA, Turner CT. An analysis of personal and social factors influencing initiation and duration of breastfeeding in a large Queensland maternity hospital. *Breastfeed Rev* 2000;8(1):25-33.

23. Bick DE, MacArthur C, Lancashire RJ. What influences the uptake and early cessation of breast feeding? *Midwifery* 1998;14(4):242-7.
24. Misri S, Sinclair DA, Kuan AJ. Breast-feeding and postpartum depression: is there a relationship? *Can J Psychiatry* 1997;42(10):1061-5.
25. Whichelow MJ. Breast feeding in Cambridge, England: factors affecting the mother's milk supply. *J Adv Nurs* 1979;4(3):253-61.
26. Scott KD, Klaus PH, Klaus MH. The obstetrical and postpartum benefits of continuous support during childbirth. *J Womens Health Gend Based Med* 1999;8(10):1257-64.

Pregnancy

Summary
Breastfeeding is not contraindicated during a normal pregnancy.

Definition/cause
The cause of pregnancy is well documented in both the academic and the popular literature.

Signs and symptoms
Early signs of pregnancy include a missed period, nausea, weight gain, breast tenderness, and fatigue. If fertilization occurs before the return of the menses, a breastfeeding woman may fail to spot the most obvious early sign of pregnancy: a missed period. Breastfeeding women also report sudden onset of sore nipples and sore breasts[1] and weaning or breast refusal in the nursing baby.[2]

Pregnancy and breastfeeding
To wean or not to wean?
In many societies worldwide, pregnancy is seen as a reason to wean the older child.[3,4] Some cultures believe that pregnancy 'spoils' the milk and makes it unhealthy for the older baby; others believe breastfeeding can harm the mother. In western cultures also, breastfeeding throughout pregnancy is an unusual event; physicians often routinely recommend rapid weaning of the older child.[4] In fact,

no studies have demonstrated that breastfeeding during pregnancy poses any risk to either the mother or unborn child,[3] and in the normal healthy pregnancy, no apparent medical reason exists for weaning. It is known however, that nipple stimulation can stimulate uterine contractions. In a high risk pregnancy, where early delivery is a concern, an obstetrician may caution against breastfeeding for this reason.

Considerations

The pregnant nursing mother will need to consider whether to wean during pregnancy, or whether to continue breastfeeding throughout the pregnancy, then to continue breastfeeding both children after the new baby is born ('tandem nursing'). The milk will revert to colostrum prior to the birth.[4] If the mother chooses to tandem nurse, the newborn should nurse before the older child in order to ensure that the new baby gets enough milk.

The older baby may wean spontaneously during pregnancy: one study of 503 women found that 69% of children who were nursing when the mother became pregnant weaned themselves before the new baby was born.[2] This may or may not be related to changes in milk composition and volume during pregnancy. Another study of two pregnant, lactating women found that milk production decreased, and breastmilk concentrations of sodium and total protein increased during pregnancy, while concentrations of potassium, glucose and lactose decreased. Changes in milk volume and composition were not significantly correlated with suckling frequency; the authors concluded that milk production decreased during pregnancy despite the positive stimulus provided by the older infant's suckling.[5]

Another study looked at 57 pregnant, breastfeeding women, of whom 43% continued to nurse throughout pregnancy, and went on to tandem nurse. Most mothers who initiated weaning cited breast and/or nipple pain as the principal reason. Most child-led weaning happened during the second trimester, and appeared to correspond with a decrease in milk supply. Infants born to the women studied were healthy and appropriate for gestational age.[1]

References
1. Moscone SR, Moore MJ. Breastfeeding during pregnancy. *J Hum Lact* 1993;9(2):83-8.

2. Newton N, Theotokatos M. Breast-feeding during pregnancy in 503 women: does psychobiological weaning mechanism exist in humans? *Emotional Reprod* 1979;20B:845.
3. Riordan J, Auerbach KG. *Breastfeeding and Human Lactation.* 2nd ed. Sudbury: Jones and Bartlett, 1999:331-32.
4. Lawrence RA, Lawrence RM. *Breastfeeding: A Guide for the Medical Profession.* 5th ed. St. Louis: Mosby; 1999:671-73.
5. Prosser CG, Saint L, Hartmann PE. Mammary gland function during gradual weaning and early gestation in women. *Aust J Exp Biol Med Sci* 1984;62(Pt 2):215-28.

Prematurity

Summary
The benefits of breastmilk are even more crucial for premature infants than for term infants. The mother of a preterm baby who wishes to breastfeed will need practical and emotional support from clinicians and hospital staff.

Definition/cause
An infant born before 37 weeks of gestational age is considered premature. Viability for premature infants begins at around 24 weeks gestation and 500g.[1] In industrialized nations, survival of infants weighing between 500 and 1000g is approximately 75%, and survival of infants weighing between 1000 and 1500g is around 90%.[2] Infants are categorized by weight as extremely low birthweight (ELBW) (below 800g); very low birthweight (VLBW) (800-1500g); and low birthweight (LBW) (1500-2500g).

A wide range of factors relating to both mothers and infants can cause premature birth.

Signs and symptoms
When compared with term infants, premature infants are small, underweight, and thin, lacking the fat stores laid down in the final weeks of pregnancy. Other signs of prematurity include lanugo, immature genitalia, and opaque or translucent skin.

Treatment

In industrialized nations, most infants born before 36 weeks gestational age are hospitalized in a Neonatal Intensive Care Unit (NICU) or in a transitional unit where they receive special care. Some stable infants around 35 weeks of gestational age may be discharged home, but feeding these often sleepy, inevitably small infants can be challenging. Breastfeeding mothers of discharged '35-36 weekers' will need extra lactation support, and may well need an electric pump at home to help stimulate milk supply.   Careful follow up of these almost-term babies is warranted.

Hospitalized premature infants usually remain in the NICU until their approximate due date.   Thus, a baby born at 28 weeks gestational age will probably remain in the NICU for about three months.

'Treatment' involves maintaining the infant in a stable condition, in an environment that imitates the dark, warm, quiet, and secure environment of the womb.   In the contemporary NICU, incubators are covered to block bright light, a quiet atmosphere is maintained, and (because premature infants have been observed to 'migrate' into the corner of the incubator), infants are surrounded by a soft buffer, not placed in the middle of an empty space.   At the same time, the infant is closely monitored for heart rate and oxygen saturation.   The major challenges involve protecting the infant from infection, preventing respiratory distress, GI obstruction, and intraventricular hemorrhage and promoting optimum growth at a rate which ideally mimics that achieved in utero.

One low-tech 'treatment' for preterm babies is kangaroo, or skin-to-skin, care.   Developed in Bogota, Columbia as an alternative to one hospital's overcrowded, understaffed special care baby unit, kangaroo care originally involved holding the stable premature infant between the mother's breasts, 24 hours a day, in a semi-upright position, for weeks or months until the infant reached around 40 weeks gestational age.   Small infants were often discharged early under this system.[2] In controlled trials of the same program in another Columbian hospital, kangaroo infants discharged early fared better than their hospital-bound peers.[3]

In nations where NICUs are well equipped with reliable life support machinery, kangaroo care has been modified to involve the infant being positioned skin-to-skin on the parent's chest, wearing only a diaper, and covered for warmth. Because the most stressful part of the procedure is moving the baby, the infant usually remains in this modified kangaroo position for at least one hour. This modified kangaroo care has been positively associated with enhanced mother-infant bonding;[4] and seen to increase oxygen saturation levels.[5] It has also been associated with increased milk production,[5,6] and longer duration of breastfeeding among NICU mothers.[5]

Prematurity and breastfeeding
Benefits of breastmilk
Clinical studies reveal that breastmilk is vital for these fragile, high-risk infants. Human milk protects against a host of infections; most significantly against necrotizing enterocolitis (NEC), an often fatal illness that targets premature infants. For preterm babies born before 30 weeks gestational age, breastmilk provides six to ten fold protection against NEC. For premies born between 30 and 37 weeks' gestational age, breastmilk provides 20 fold protection, when compared to formula-fed preterm babies.[7,8]

Breastmilk also protects premature infants against intestinal and respiratory tract infections,[7] aids digestion and absorption of nutrients, assists gastrointestinal function, and protects against sepsis and meningitis.[8,9] It improves visual function[10,11] and appears to enhance neurocognitive development.[12,13] Premature infants fed human milk have also been shown to have faster brainstem maturation when compared to formula-fed infants.[14] The milk of mothers whose babies are born preterm contains more protein, nitrogen, fatty acids, sodium, chloride, iron, zinc, and magnesium than the milk of mothers whose infants are born at term.

The act of breastfeeding for premature infants capable of feeding by mouth is less stressful than bottle-feeding. Oxygen saturation and body temperature remains higher during breastfeeding than during bottle-feeding, and infants are less likely to desaturate to 90% oxygen during breastfeeding.[15]

The benefits of breastmilk for these babies are overwhelming; however, the prospect of providing milk for a NICU infant can also be overwhelming, and hospital support for these mothers is crucial.

Breastfeeding a premature baby: practical aspects and support

Because most premature infants are too small or weak to nurse at the breast, the mother will need a top quality, double setup electric breast pump (see Breastfeeding aids) as soon as practical after birth, on the postpartum unit, to stimulate the breasts and initiate milk production. Frequency of pumping is always a balance between the ideal and the practical, but the research-based standard recommends double pumping, at least five times in 24 hours, for a total pumping time of approximately 100 minutes per day,[16] until the baby is able to nurse directly at the breast. Practically, this usually translates into double pumping approximately every three hours for 10-15 minutes, around the clock.

Approaching the NICU mother about breastfeeding requires tact and optimism. Clearly, she is under a great deal of stress, and may never have considered using an electric breast pump. Indeed, she may never even have considered breastfeeding. Given the benefits of breastmilk for the premature infant, the clinician should inform the mother of this option for her child, and dispel any fears she may have about the appropriateness of her milk, and her ability to supply milk under these conditions. Some mothers may choose only to pump for the few days they spend in hospital, which is a valid option. Other women pump for months and find great comfort in knowing there is something practical and useful that they alone can do for their high-risk infant amid the overwhelming numbers of wires, monitors, and machines.

All mothers will require encouragement during the first few pumping episodes; some women may see no milk at all during the first 24 hours, even if they pump religiously every three hours. Other women may see only small quantities of colostrum. Because colostrum may be clear or yellow, some women assume this is not 'real' milk (some believe it is water) and may be tempted to discard it, especially when only very small amounts are pumped. Telling the mother that this is 'liquid gold' filled with beneficial nutrients, and reminding her that her premature baby requires only very small amounts at each feed will reassure her of the value of her early milk. On discharge, the breastfeeding NICU mother will need a top quality breast pump at home (see Breastfeeding aids).

184

Ideally, the premature infant's first oral feeding experience should be at the breast. Often the infant is first put to breast while tube feeds are given via the nose, and thus learns to associate the breast with feeding. Initially the infant should show some interest in the nipple, and may root, open the mouth, lick, and attempt to latch. Even when the infant nurses well, s/he may tire easily, and the mother should be reassured that this is normal at early oral feeds. Eventually, most infants are able to feed entirely at the breast.

Overcoming problems

Common problems for NICU mothers include a dwindling milk supply over time, feelings of guilt, stress and exhaustion, and disappointment if the infant's early attempts to feed at the breast are unsuccessful. A less common problem can be over-supply with a tendency to engorgement, plugged ducts, and mastitis, especially if women pump too frequently or for too long at each pumping session. Strategies to increase milk supply include increasing the frequency of pumping, ensuring that the mother is using a top quality pump, and using kangaroo or 'skin-to-skin' care.[17]   If these methods prove unsuccessful, numerous studies indicate that the medication metoclopramide (Reglan), which is usually used to treat gastroesophageal reflux, will increase milk supply in most lactating women with inadequate supply.[18-20]   Fenugreek is a popularly recommended herbal treatment for increasing milk supply. (See Low milk supply).

Over-supply can be treated with conventional engorgement therapies (see Engorgement), less frequent pumping, or shortened duration of pumping.

References

1.   Lawrence RA, Lawrence RM. *Breastfeeding: A Guide for the Medical Profession.* 5th ed. St. Louis: Mosby; 1999:443-467.
2.   Whitelaw A, Sleath K. Myth of the marsupial mother: home care of very low birth weight babies in Bogota, Colombia. *Lancet* 1985;1(8439):1206-8.
3.   Charpak N, Ruiz-Pelaez JG, Figueroa de CZ, Charpak Y. Kangaroo mother versus traditional care for newborn infants /=2000 grams: a randomized, controlled trial. *Pediatrics* 1997;100(4):682-8.

4. Tessier R, Cristo M, Velez S, Giron M, de Calume ZF, Ruiz-Palaez JG, et al. Kangaroo mother care and the bonding hypothesis. *Pediatrics* 1998;102(2):e17.
5. Bier JA, Ferguson AE, Morales Y, Liebling JA, Archer D, Oh W, et al. Comparison of skin-to-skin contact with standard contact in low-birth-weight infants who are breast-fed. *Arch Pediatr Adolesc Med* 1996;150(12):1265-9.
6. Schanler RJ, Hurst NM, Lau C. The use of human milk and breastfeeding in premature infants. *Clin Perinatol* 1999;26(2):379-98, vii.
7. Lucas A, Cole TJ. Breast milk and neonatal necrotising enterocolitis. *Lancet* 1990;336(8730):1519-23.
8. Schanler RJ, Shulman RJ, Lau C. Feeding strategies for premature infants: beneficial outcomes of feeding fortified human milk versus preterm formula. *Pediatrics* 1999;103(6 Pt 1):1150-7.
9. Hylander MA, Strobino DM, Dhanireddy R. Human milk feedings and infection among very low birth weight infants. *Pediatrics* 1998;102(3):E38.
10. Hylander MA ea. Human milk feedings and retinopathy of prematurity (ROP) among very low birth weight (VLBW) infants. *Pediatr Res* 1995;37:214a.
11. Birch E, Birch D, Hoffman D, Hale L, Everett M, Uauy R. Breast-feeding and optimal visual development. *J Pediatr Ophthalmol Strabismus* 1993;30(1):33-8.
12. Lucas A, Morley R, Cole TJ, Lister G, Leeson-Payne C. Breast milk and subsequent intelligence quotient in children born preterm. *Lancet* 1992;339(8788):261-4.
13. Morley R, Cole TJ, Powell R, Lucas A. Mother's choice to provide breast milk and developmental outcome. *Arch Dis Child* 1988;63(11):1382-5.
14. Amin SB, Merle KS, Orlando MS, Dalzell LE, Guillet R. Brainstem maturation in premature infants as a function of enteral feeding type. *Pediatrics* 2000;106(2 Pt 1):318-22.
15. Blaymore Bier JA, Ferguson AE, Morales Y, Liebling JA, Oh W, Vohr BR. Breastfeeding infants who were extremely low birth weight. *Pediatrics* 1997;100(6):E3.
16. Hopkinson JM, Schanler RJ, Garza C. Milk production by mothers of premature infants. *Pediatrics* 1988;81(6):815-20.
17. Anderson GC. Current knowledge about skin-to-skin (kangaroo) care for preterm infants. *J Perinatol* 1991;11(3):216-26.
18. Kauppila A, Kivinen S, Ylikorkala O. A dose response relation between improved lactation and metoclopramide. *Lancet* 1981;1(8231):1175-7.

19. Ehrenkranz RA, Ackerman BA. Metoclopramide effect on faltering milk production by mothers of premature infants. *Pediatrics* 1986;78(4):614-20.
20. Guzman V, Toscano G, Canales ES, Zarate A. Improvement of defective lactation by using oral metoclopramide. *Acta Obstet Gynecol Scand* 1979;58(1):53-5.

Primary dysmenorrhea (Menstrual cramps)

Summary
Women with primary dysmenorrhea can breastfeed.
Definition/cause
Primary dysmenorrhea is a symptom complex which includes colicky menstrual cramps occurring at the onset of menstruation and potentially several days into the period. The condition is associated with ovulatory cycles, and without other ongoing pelvic disorders. It is caused by the activity of prostaglandins PGE_2 and PGF_2 , which are produced locally by the endometrium, and stimulate uterine contractions causing hypoxia, ischemia, and pain.[1]

Signs and symptoms
The onset of the menstrual period is associated with painful abdominal cramps, and possibly with nausea, vomiting, diarrhea, backache, headache, and general malaise.

Treatment
Either at, or shortly before the onset of menses, the affected individual can take nonsteroidal anti-inflammatory drugs (NSAIDs) which inhibit prostaglandin activity.[2,3] NSAIDs include ibuprofen, naproxen, naproxen sodium, or mefenamic acid. If this first line of defense does not work, oral contraceptives may be prescribed. Contraceptives are believed to effectively treat primary dysmenorrhea by preventing ovulation and by provoking endometrial hypoplasia, thus keeping prostaglandin levels low.[4,5]

Primary dysmenorrhea and breastfeeding
Women with primary dysmenorrhea can breastfeed. However, if birth control pills are recommended as therapy, estrogen-containing

pills should be avoided, because estrogen has been shown to reduce milk supply in lactating women.[6] Progestin-only birth control pills can effectively control the pain of primary dysmenorrhea, and do not appear to reduce milk supply.[7]

The return of menses following birth varies widely from woman to woman. Wang cites an average of eight to 15 months amenorrhea among lactating women, compared to about two months in non-breastfeeding women, although some breastfeeding women menstruate earlier than this.[8] In breastfeeding women, the return of fertility and the first ovulation is influenced by breastfeeding frequency, and not just by the return of menses.[8,9] Anovular first periods are common.[9,10]

Food for thought
- Dysmenorrhea is Greek for 'difficult monthly flow'.
- Vane and his co-researchers were awarded the Nobel prize for discovering that NSAIDs work by inhibiting prostaglandin synthetase, the enzyme responsible for the creation of prostaglandins.[2,3]

References
1. Alvin PE, Litt IF. Current status of the etiology and management of dysmenorrhea in adolescence. *Pediatrics* 1982;70(4):516-25.
2. Vane J. Inhibition of prostaglandin synthesis as a mechnism of action of aspirin-like drugs. *Nature New Biol* 1971;234:231-238.
3. Ferreira S, Vane J. New aspects of the mode of action of nonsteroidal anti-inflammatory drugs. *Annu Rev Pharm* 1974;14:57-73.
4. Simon LS, Mills JA. Drug therapy: nonsteroidal antiinflammatory drugs (first of two parts). *N Engl J Med* 1980;302(21):1179-85.
5. Simon LS, Mills JA. Nonsteroidal anti-inflammatory drugs (second of two parts). *N Engl J Med* 1980;302(22):1237-43.
6. Hale TW. *Medications and Mothers' Milk*. 9th ed. Amarillo: Pharmasoft Publishing, 2000:242.
7. Dunson TR, McLaurin VL, Grubb GS, Rosman AW. A multicenter clinical trial of a progestin-only oral contraceptive in lactating women. *Contraception* 1993;47(1):23-35.
8. Wang IY, Fraser IS. Reproductive function and contraception in the postpartum period. *Obstet Gynecol Surv* 1994;49(1):56-63.
9. Gray RH, Campbell OM, Apelo R, Eslami SS, Zacur H, Ramos RM, et al. Risk of ovulation during lactation. *Lancet* 1990;335(8680):25-9.

10. Eslami SS, Gray RH, Apelo R, Ramos R. The reliability of menses to indicate the return of ovulation in breastfeeding women in Manila, The Philippines. *Stud Fam Plann* 1990;21(5):243-50.

Psoriasis

Summary
Women with psoriasis can breastfeed, but their type of therapy may be of concern.

Definition/cause
Psoriasis is a chronic skin disease, the cause of which is unknown, although there appears to be a familial tendency towards it. Affecting 1-3% of the US population, it is more common in whites than blacks, and rare in Asians and Native Americans.[1] In 10% of cases psoriasis develops by age 10, and in 35% of cases it develops by age 20;[2] the ratio for female:male is 2:1 when the disease develops before age 16.

In psoriasis, an abnormally rapid turnover of the epidermis occurs. The condition is marked by unpredictable periods of remission and exacerbation. Certain factors can cause or worsen the characteristic skin eruptions; these include physical trauma, stress, sunburn, certain medications (such as lithium and beta blockers), and infections.

Signs and symptoms
Psoriasis is characterized by red, scaly lesions, which commonly occur on the scalp, chest, elbows, knees, extensor surfaces of the limbs, lower back, buttocks, and genitalia. The lesions begin as small, red papules topped by fine scales. The papules combine to form varied numbers of well-marginated plaques, which are often distributed bilaterally and symmetrically, and vary in size and severity from individual to individual. The silver-white (mica-like) scales are attached at the center, rather than the periphery of the lesion; when the scale is removed it leaves a fine bleeding point known as Auspitz's sign. The appearance of lesions at the site of skin damage (caused,

for example, by surgery, abrasions, bites, burns, skin tests, vaccinations, or venipuncture) is known as Koebner's phenomenon. Nail involvement, most commonly pitting, is seen in 25-50% of affected individuals, and psoriatic arthritis occurs in 5-10% of cases. Psoriasis can affect the breast or nipple.[3]

Treatment

Treatment depends on the type, extent, and location of the lesions.   Therapies aim to reduce irritation and to control skin lesions; there is no cure for psoriasis per se.   The most effective therapy appears to be exposure to sunlight;[2]   most patients improve in the summer time.   Other treatments include exposure to ultraviolet B spectrum of light, alone or in combination with coal tar or anthralin; topical agents including tar preparations and topical vitamin D analogs; and systemic medications such as methotrexate and retinoids.

Steroids are generally not recommended because the disease rebounds after their use.[4]

Psoriasis medications and breastfeeding

A thorough review of treatment options and their significance for breastfeeding women is presented in Hale's *Clinical Therapy in Breastfeeding Patients*.[4]

Topical steroids are no longer routinely recommended for treatment of psoriasis,[4]   thus questions on their use in this skin condition should not arise.   Anthralin is commonly prescribed: little is absorbed systemically after topical use,[4] but if possible, the mother should avoid intensive, widespread use during breastfeeding, and avoid direct use on the nipples.   If she must use it on the nipple, temporary cessation of breastfeeding on the affected breast may be necessary, although the baby can continue to nurse on the unaffected side, and the mother can pump the other breast to maintain milk supply.   If retinoids are needed, etretinate should be avoided, but tazarotene, which is poorly absorbed through the skin, is unlikely to affect the breastfeeding baby.[4]

Psoriasis and breastfeeding

It is the medications used to treat psoriasis which may create problems for breastfeeding women, rather than the presence of the disease itself (see above).

Food for thought

- A variety of psoriasis, gluttate psoriasis, is most commonly seen in children and young adults, and often presents after a group A streptococcal infection.

Reference

1. Nigro JF, Esterly NB. Psoriasis - chronic but controllable. *Cont Peds* 1993(October):114-130.
2. Johnson KB, Oski FA. *Oski's Essential Pediatrics.* 2nd ed. Philadelphia:Lippincott and Raven; 1997:119.
3. Stern RS. Psoriasis. *Lancet* 1997;350(9074):349-53.
4. Hale TW. *Clinical Therapy in Breastfeeding Patients.* Amarillo:Pharmasoft Publishing; 1999:149-51.

Pyloric stenosis

Summary

The infant with pyloric stenosis can breastfeed as tolerated before and after surgery.

Definition/cause

Pyloric stenosis is caused by hypertrophy of the pyloric muscle, resulting in an obstruction of fluids passing from the stomach to the small intestine. It is the most common condition requiring surgery in the early months of life,[1] and is believed to develop postnatally, although the precise cause is unknown. The only reliably consistent associations appear to be family history, and a preponderance of pyloric stenosis among first born infants[2-4] and males[3,5,6].

Signs and symptoms

Pyloric stenosis usually presents in the first three months of life with non-bilious projectile vomiting, which occurs initially after some feeds, and eventually after every feed. The parent often describes the vomit as forceful, "shooting across the room." It is markedly different from the occasional dribbling or spitting up that is normal in young infants. Initially, infants with pyloric stenosis are hungry and go back for more food, but with recurrent vomiting they become fussy, irritable, and weak, with decreased urine and stool output, eventually losing weight and becoming dehydrated. By contrast, an infant vomiting from overfeeding will gain weight and thrive. Electrolyte imbalance reflects chronic loss of gastric fluids: a hypochloremia metabolic alkalosis.

On examination, the thickened pyloric muscle may be palpable as an 'olive-like' mass in the right upper quadrant of the abdomen, near the midline. Ultrasound will accurately reveal a thickened and elongated pyloric muscle in 90% of cases.

Treatment

Surgery, specifically a pyloromyotomy, corrects the problem. Preoperatively, it is imperative to correct any fluid and electrolyte imbalance. As the infant is often incapable of keeping down fluid at this point, rehydration is usually intravenous.

Pyloric stenosis and breastfeeding

As with many other factors surrounding pyloric stenosis, its association with feeding method is unclear. Three studies suggest possible decreased rate of pyloric stenosis in breastfed infants,[3,5,7] but other studies found that the feeding method was irrelevant to the incidence of the condition.[6,8] During the surgical period, and until the infant is able to tolerate oral feeds, the mother should acquire a good quality electric breast pump and pump her breasts- approximately every three hours for 10-15 minutes - to maintain a milk supply. Any pumped milk can be stored and given later to the infant.

Food for thought

• Infants exposed prenatally to thalidomide have a high incidence of pyloric stenosis.[9]

References
1. Ohshiro K, Puri P.   Pathogenesis of infantile hypertrophic pyloric stenosis: recent progress. *Pediatr Surg Int* 1998;13(4):243-52.

2. Jedd MB, Melton LJd, Griffin MR, Kaufman B, Hoffman AD, Broughton D, et al. Factors associated with infantile hypertrophic pyloric stenosis. *Am J Dis Child* 1988;142(3):334-7.
3. Webb AR, Lari J, Dodge JA. Infantile hypertrophic pyloric stenosis in South Glamorgan 1970-9. Effects of changes in feeding practice. *Arch Dis Child* 1983;58(8):586-90.
4. Dodge JA. Infantile hypertrophic pyloric stenosis in Belfast, 1957-1969. *Arch Dis Child* 1975;50(3):171-8.
5. Habbick BF, Khanna C, To T. Infantile hypertrophic pyloric stenosis: a study of feeding practices and other possible causes. *Cmaj* 1989;140(4):401-4.
6. Lammer EJ, Edmonds LD. Trends in pyloric stenosis incidence, Atlanta, 1968 to 1982. *J Med Genet* 1987;24(8):482-7.
7. Pisacane A, de Luca U, Criscuolo L, Vaccaro F, Valiante A, Inglese A, et al. Breast feeding and hypertrophic pyloric stenosis: population based case-control study. *BMJ* 1996;312(7033):745-6.
8. Hitchcock NE, Gilmour AI, Gracey M, Burke V. Pyloric stenosis in Western Australia, 1971-84. *Arch Dis Child* 1987;62(5):512-3.
9. Schafer KH, Kramer M. Infantile hypertrophic pyloric stenosis after prenatal exposure to thalidomide. *Eur J Pediatr* 1987;146(1):63-7.

Rabies

Summary

If the mother is exposed to rabies, she can continue breastfeeding after she receives immune globulin and begins the vaccination series.

Definition/cause

Rabies is an acute, rapidly progressing, usually lethal illness caused by a RNA-containing virus that can affect any warm-blooded animal. Commonly infected mammals that may come into contact with human beings include raccoons, bats, skunks, foxes, coyotes, cats, dogs, ferrets, and, as rabies becomes established in particular regions, domesticated livestock. Transmission from small rodents to human beings is rare. Because the incubation period is usually four to six weeks, and can last up to six years, the source of rabies in some individuals can be unknown.[1]

The disease is usually transmitted when an infected animal bites a human being and deposits virus-laden saliva into the open wound.[2,3] The virus multiplies locally and reaches the peripheral nerves, progressing to the spinal cord and central nervous system. Death usually occurs within ten days of initial symptoms.

Only 36 deaths from rabies occurred in the US between 1980 and 1996, although many more people were vaccinated after suspected exposure. Worldwide, rabies accounts for 40,000-100,000 deaths per year.

Signs and symptoms

Initial symptoms are non-specific: fever, headache, malaise and gastrointestinal upset, with pain or paresthesia (numbness) at the site of the bite. During the neurologic stage, symptoms include aggressive, bizarre behaviors such as hyperactivity, agitation, anxiety, hydrophobia, and seizures. Half of victims suffer from dysphagia and hypersalivation. The disease progresses rapidly to encephalitis, followed by a comatose state, possible paralysis, and death.[2,3]

Treatment

If a suspicious, high risk bite occurs, the wound should immediately be thoroughly washed with soap and water. If available, the animal should be destroyed and the brain sent to be analyzed for possible rabies infection. The bite victim should immediately receive human rabies immune globulin (HRIG) and begin the five dose vaccination series (IM injections on days 0,3,7,14, and 28). One-half of the immune globulin is injected directly into the wound and the other half into the buttock. If the animal brain biopsy proves negative, the vaccination series can be stopped.[1]

Human rabies is best prevented by avoiding contact with rabid animals and by decreasing the pool of rabid animals through mass immunization programs targeting both wild and domestic animals. Veterinarians and others at high risk of rabies exposure should receive pre-exposure prophylaxis of a three dose vaccination series.[1]

Rabies and breastfeeding

Person to person transmission of rabies has not been reliably documented except for case reports involving corneal transplants. Neither is there any reliable documentation of transmission of the rabies virus reported through breastmilk.[4,5]   If a nursing mother encounters a possible rabies source, she should immediately receive the human rabies immune globulin and begin the vaccination series. Breastfeeding may continue once this has started; rabies vaccine is prepared from inactivated rabies virus and there is no reason to believe it would have any untoward effect on the nursing infant.[6] If the animal is negative for rabies, the vaccination series can be stopped.

Food for thought
- Hawaii is the only rabies-free state in the US.
- The islands of Australia, Great Britain, and Ireland are rabies-free.
- Rabies prophylaxis costs approximately US $1,500 per patient.[7]

Resources
Rabies advice is available from rabies section of the Centers for Disease Control and Prevention: Tel. 404-639-1050/1075.

References
1.   American Academy of Pediatrics. In: Pickering LK, ed. *2000 Red Book: Report of the Committee on Infectious Diseases.* 25th ed. Elk Grove Village, IL: American Academy of Pediatrics;2000:475-482.
2.   Schmidt MJ, Olson JG, Krebs JW.   Rabies goes wild. *Contemporary Ped* 1993;August:36-46.
3.   Phelps R.   Rabies: Confronting the continuing threat. *Contemporary Ped* 1997;14(7):136-150.
4.   Lawrence RA, Lawrence RM. *Breastfeeding: a Guide for the Medical Profession.* 5th ed. St. Louis: Mosby; 1999:604-5.
5.   Hall TG, ed. *Diseases Transmitted from Animal to Man.* Springfield, Il: Thomas 1963; 293-7.
6.   Hale TW.   *Medications and Mothers' Milk.* 9th ed. Amarillo: Pharmasoft Publishing; 1999:571.
7.   Prophylaxis for rabies off base. *Pediatric News* Nov 2000; 34 (11):10.

Reactive airway disease (Asthma)

Summary

A mother or infant with reactive airway disease can breastfeed.

Definition/cause

Reactive airway disease is a common, sometimes chronic, inflammatory airway disorder that describes varying degrees of diffuse, obstructive lung disease. Where only one or two episodes of wheezing are recorded in the young infant, the condition may simply be called 'wheezing'. The terms reactive airway disease and asthma, tend to be applied when the condition manifests as chronic. The airway obstruction can be caused by *inflammation* of the bronchial wall and the surrounding tissue causing edema, infiltration of cells and desquamation of cells into the lumen; *mucous production* within the airway; or *bronchoconstriction* due to smooth muscle contraction. The end result is a narrow, plugged airway.

In western nations, up to 10% of the pediatric population under 16 years of age may be affected. In childhood asthma, 20-30% of patients develop symptoms within the first year of life, with the average age of onset being four years.[1] Since the 1970s, the prevalence of asthma has been increasing in the United States, particularly among urban populations of low socioeconomic status. In 60% of cases, childhood asthma resolves by young adult life.

The disease is characterized by hyperreactivity of bronchi to various stimuli or triggers, and airflow obstruction, which either reverses spontaneously or in response to treatment. Common triggers include viral infections that cause upper respiratory tract infections, animals (especially cats and dogs), molds, dust mites, cockroaches, pollens, changes in the weather or cold weather, and cigarette smoke.

Signs and symptoms

The course and severity of asthmatic attacks are highly variable. Symptoms include cough (initially tight and non-productive), wheezing, shortness of breath, elevated respiratory rate, a prolonged expiratory phase, use of accessory muscles of respiration, cyanosis,

196

respiratory distress, and hyperinflation of the chest. Affected individuals may cough up mucous plugs.

Treatment

Patients should be educated about the chronic nature of the disease, and avoid personal triggers. Therapy depends on the severity, which can be classified as mild and intermittent; mild and persistent; moderate and persistent, or severe and persistent.[2]

Asthma medications and breastfeeding

An in-depth review of asthma medications and breastfeeding is available in Hale's *Clinical Therapy in Breastfeeding Patients*.[3] Generally, medications for asthmatics are compatible with breastfeeding. Asthma is an inflammatory disease, hence anti-inflammatory corticosteroids such as beclomethasone, flunisolide, fluticasone, triamcinolone acetonide, budesonide, and methylprednisolone constitute the most potent treatments. Both maternal plasma levels, and transfer of these corticosteroids into human milk is low and unlikely to be of concern in breastfeeding women.[3] Beta adrenergic agonists, such as albuterol and terbutaline, which work by affecting beta 2 receptors on bronchial smooth muscle to cause bronchodilatation, are also used. Levels in breastmilk are low and not believed to be of concern.[3] Mast cell stabilizers like cromolyn sodium may also prove effective; cromolyn is not orally bioavailable to the breastfeeding infant because it is not systemically absorbed by the mother.[3]

Reactive airway disease and breastfeeding

Women or infants with reactive airway disease can breastfeed, and parents with a family history of asthma should be strongly encouraged to breastfeed exclusively whenever possible, because of the long term protective effect of breastfeeding on asthma.[4-8]

One trial of 453 children with a family history of allergic disease found that children who had been breastfed had a lower incidence of wheeze than those who had not, and that at age seven, the risk of wheezing was halved in the breastfed children.[4] A study by Oddy followed 2187 Australian children and found that exclusive breastfeeding for four months of age resulted in a significant reduction in the risk of childhood asthma at age six.[5]

Resources
Asthma and Allergy Foundation of America
1233 20th St., NW Ste. 402
Washington DC 20036
800/727-8462
202/466-7643
info@aafa.org

References
1. McMillan JA, DeAngelis CD, Feigin RD, Warshaw JB eds. *Oski's Pediatrics:Principles and Practice.* 3rd ed. Philadelphia:Lippincourt Williams and Wilkins;1999:2041-2048.
2. National Heart, Lung and Blood Institute. National Asthma Education and Prevention Program. Guidelines for diagnosis and management of asthma. Publication #97-4051. Bethesda, MD: National Institutes of Health, 1997.
3. Hale TW. *Clinical Therapy in Breastfeeding Patients.* 1st ed. Amarillo:Pharmasoft Medical Publishing; 1999.
4. Burr ML, Limb ES, Maguire MJ, Amarah L, Eldridge BA, Layzell JC, et al. Infant feeding, wheezing, and allergy: a prospective study. *Arch Dis Child* 1993;68(6):724-8.
5. Oddy WH, Holt PG, Sly PD, Read AW, Landau LI, Stanley FJ, et al. Association between breast feeding and asthma in 6 year old children: findings of a prospective birth cohort study. *BMJ* 1999;319(7213):815-9.
6. Miskelly FG, Burr ML, Vaughan-Williams E, Fehily AM, Butland BK, Merrett TG. Infant feeding and allergy. *Arch Dis Child* 1988;63(4):388-93.
7. Chandra RK. Five-year follow-up of high-risk infants with family history of allergy who were exclusively breast-fed or fed partial whey hydrolysate, soy, and conventional cow's milk formulas. *J Pediatr Gastroenterol Nutr* 1997;24(4):380-8.
8. Romieu I, Werneck G, Ruiz Velasco S, White M, Hernandez M. Breastfeeding and asthma among Brazilian children. *J Asthma* 2000;37(7):575-83.

Reduction mammoplasty (Breast reduction surgery)

Summary

Women who have undergone reduction mammoplasty should be encouraged to breastfeed. However, some women cannot produce enough milk: the mother should be counseled appropriately and the infant's weight should be carefully monitored.

Definition/cause

Surgery to reduce breast size, whether for cosmetic reasons or, in some cases, to relieve back pain, is usually done by one of two methods.

The 'pedicle' technique leaves the nipple and areola attached to the breast during surgery, while tissue is removed from beneath and the sides of the breast. Successful breastfeeding has been described after the use of this technique, although supplementation is sometimes necessary.[1-4]

The 'free nipple' technique involves periareolar surgery, with complete removal of the nipple and areola, which are stitched back onto the breast following removal of tissue. Because the nerves, blood vessels, and milk ducts are severed during this process, women who undergo this type of surgery are more likely to have breastfeeding problems.[2,5]

Signs and symptoms

Usually a women will self-report if she has had breast surgery, but a clinician should perform a breast exam, ideally during the prenatal period, on any woman planning to breastfeed, and look for surgical scars, as well as for other potential complications. Because different types of surgery can affect lactation in differing ways, it is important to establish why the surgery was performed and, if possible, what technique was used.

Reduction mammoplasty and breastfeeding

Women who have undergone reduction mammoplasty should be encouraged to breastfeed if they so desire. Studies show that health care professionals may dissuade these women from nursing, and that many of them do not attempt breastfeeding as a result.[6]   In Brzozowski's study, 27 of 78 women who had children postoperatively were discouraged from breastfeeding by medical professionals, and only eight of the 27 (29.6% percent) subsequently tried to breastfeed. By comparison, 26 patients were encouraged to breastfeed and 19 (73.1%) of them subsequently attempted breastfeeding.[1]

Women who have had breast reduction surgery, especially periareolar surgery where the nipple and areola were completely removed, may not produce a full milk supply. In one study, women with periareolar breast incisions were nearly five times more likely to have lactation insufficiency than women without surgery.[5]

However, Brzozowski found that among 78 patients who had breast reduction surgery using the pedicle technique, 15 (19.2% percent) breastfed exclusively, eight (10.3%) breastfed with formula supplementation, and 14 (17.9%) attempted breastfeeding without success.   The remaining 41 women (52.6 percent) did not attempt breastfeeding.[1]

While encouraging the mother to breastfeed, therefore, the clinician should be sure that she is aware of the possibility of not producing enough milk.   Some signs of potential problems include lack of sensation in the nipple (indicating severed nerve ducts), and older surgeries, especially if breastfeeding was not discussed with the surgeon.   The mother may lactate successfully in the hospital, producing adequate colostrum, but her milk may not fully 'come in', or she may not be able to keep up with the demands of a growing baby. The baby should have an early weight check, and weight gain and stool patterns should be closely monitored.   If the mother wishes to continue feeding at breast, but is unable to produce an adequate milk supply, she may choose to use a Supplemental Nursing System™ (see Breastfeeding aids).

References

1.   Brzozowski D, Niessen M, Evans HB, Hurst LN. Breast-feeding after inferior pedicle reduction mammaplasty. *Plast Reconstr Surg* 2000;105(2):530-4.
2.   Marshall DR, Callan PP, Nicholson W. Breastfeeding after reduction mammaplasty. *Br J Plast Surg* 1994;47(3):167-9.

3. Harris L, Morris SF, Freiberg A.   Is breast feeding possible after reduction mammaplasty? *Plast Reconstr Surg* 1992;89(5):836-9.
4. Caouette-Laberge L, Duranceau LA.   Breast feeding after breast reduction. *Ann Chir* 1992;46(9):826-9.
5. Neifert M, DeMarzo S, Seacat J, Young D, Leff M, Orleans M.   The influence of breast surgery, breast appearance, and pregnancy- induced breast changes on lactation sufficiency as measured by infant weight gain. *Birth* 1990;17(1):31-8.
6. Deutinger M, Deutinger J.   Breast feeding following breast reduction-plasty and mastopexy? *Geburtshilfe Frauenheilkd* 1990;50(3):220-2.

Rickets

Summary

Some exclusively breastfed infants may require vitamin D supplementation to avoid development of rickets.   According to the American Academy of Pediatrics, "Vitamin D...may need to be given before six months of age in selected groups of infants....whose mothers are vitamin D-deficient or those infants not exposed to adequate sunlight."[1]

Definition/cause

Rickets occurs when the bone matrix fails to mineralize.   It is usually caused by a lack of vitamin D.

Between birth and six months, the infant receives vitamin D from diet, exposure to sunlight, and from maternal stores which have been transferred transplacentally to the fetus.   If inadequate exposure to sunlight occurs, experts recommend an infant between birth and one year receive a daily vitamin D intake of 200 IU, and comment that 400 IU per day would not be excessive.[2]

Vitamin D is essential for the maintenance of a healthy skeleton throughout life.   Vitamin D (calciferol) includes a group of fat-soluble seco-sterols, among which are vitamin D_2, vitamin D_3, and vitamin D. Human beings obtain vitamin D either by oral consumption or by cutaneous photosynthesis.   Only a few foods contain vitamin D: fish liver oils, the flesh of fatty fish, the liver and fat from aquatic mammals such as seals and polar bears, and eggs from hens that have been fed vitamin D fortified foods.   Given the general lack of these foods in the typical western diet, oral intake often comes from fortified foods, particularly milk. Vitamin D is also added to some cereals, breads and margarine. Infant formulas are vitamin-D fortified by law (400 IU/L) while rice and soy drinks are not. Breastmilk contains approximately 22-40 IU/L.

Exposure to sunlight provides humans with much of their vitamin D requirement. Vitamin D_3 is produced when 7-dehydrocholesterol, a substance found in the skin, is exposed to ultraviolet B radiation (found in the 290-320 nm range). Once formed, Vitamin D_3 enters the circulatory system via absorption into dermal capillaries. In the liver, one hydroxylation occurs, forming 25-hydroxyvitamin D or 25(OH)D.

A second hydroxylation occurs in the kidney, forming $1,25(OH)_2D$ to create the biologically active form of vitamin D.

The major function of vitamin D is to maintain the extracellular concentration of calcium (Ca) and phosphorous (P) within the normal range in one of two ways. Vitamin D enhances the efficiency of the absorption of dietary Ca and P from the small intestine. With adequate levels of vitamin D, Ca and P are maintained at supersaturating concentrations and are available for mineralization of bone. If dietary intake cannot meet the body's needs, vitamin D, along with parathyroid hormone (PTH), stimulates mobilization of Ca and P stores from bones.

Signs and symptoms

Clinical findings of rickets include deformities of the skeleton, enlargement of the wrists and ankles, enlargement of the joints of the long bones and rib cage, curvature of the spine and thighs, enlargement of the head, shortened stature, generalized muscle weakness, and abnormalities of calcium levels associated with seizures. Other specific findings can include 'craniotabes', which may be detected on physical exam by pressing the occiput or posterior parietal bones and feeling a ping-pong ball sensation due to thinning of the outer table of the skull; the characteristic 'rachitic rosary', a palpable enlargement of the costochondral junctions of the rib cage, and 'caput quadratum': the box-like appearance of the head due to the softness of the skull and subsequent flattening. 'Pigeon breast deformity' is caused by the apparent forward projection of the sternum; bow legs or knock knees are other characteristic symptoms.[3]

An x-ray of the wrist is useful for early diagnosis, because changes to the ulna and radius occur early on. The distal ends become widened, cupped and frayed, in contrast to their normal sharp delineation and convex ends, and the density of the shaft decreases.

In mild cases, biochemical findings include decreased serum calcium levels, increased parathyroid hormones, normal levels of phosphorus, and elevated levels of serum alkaline phosphatase. As disease becomes more severe, serum phosphorus levels may drop and calcium may normalize. In the most severe cases, both calcium and phosphorus levels are low, PTH and alkaline phosphatase are elevated, and levels of 25(OH)D are decreased.

Treatment

Prevention of rickets requires adequate exposure to sunlight, or vitamin D supplementation of the diet. Vitamin D supplementation for infants in the US is usually given in the most available form, which is in combination with vitamins, A and C. Both vitamins A and C are sufficient in breastmilk, but preparations of exclusive vitamin D are expensive and rarely used.

Rickets can be treated with vitamin D supplements direct to the infant. The size of the dose will depend on the severity of the condition.

Rickets and breastfeeding

The American Academy of Pediatrics has three official publications that discuss breastfeeding, rickets and sunlight exposure. In *Breastfeeding and the Use of Human Milk*, the AAP states: "Vitamin D and iron may need to be given before six months of age in selected groups of infants (vitamin D for mothers who are vitamin D deficient or those infants not exposed to adequate sunlight; iron for those who have low iron stores or anemia.)".[1] The AAP Pediatric Nutrition Handbook states: "There is little biologically active vitamin D in human milk. Therefore, dark-skinned infants will need vitamin D supplement particularly if they are exposed to minimum amounts of sunlight (pp14-15) ...Milk from a well-nourished mother contains sufficient vitamins for the young healthy term infant except for vitamin D and for vitamin K during the first few days of life (p 267)...The vitamin D content of human milk is low (22 IU/L) and rickets can occur in deeply pigmented breastfed infants or in those with inadequate exposure to sunlight. Consequently, vitamin D supplementation at 400 IU/day is recommended for breastfed infants (p 275)"[4]

Recommendations by the AAP regarding sunlight exposure in *Ultraviolet Light: A Hazard to Children* encourages protection from the sun's rays. Specifically, this publication states that "infants under six months should be kept out of direct sunlight....clothes offer the simplest and often most practical means of sun protection" and suggests that in children under six months it "may be reasonable to apply sunscreen to small areas, such as the face and the back of the hands." In addition, the AAP states, "children's activities should be selected to avoid or minimize sun exposure between 10 am and 4 pm".[5] Thus current medical wisdom encourages protecting young children from the sun; however some sunlight exposure is necessary to ensure a child's vitamin D supply.

Many other lifestyle issues can also result in inadequate sunlight exposure. The more melanin in the skin, the less efficient is the sun-mediated photosynthesis of vitamin D_3; thus dark skinned infants living in areas with limited hours of sunshine are more susceptible to vitamin D deficiency than light skinned individuals in the same climate. Similarly, individuals living in urban settings receive less sunlight than individuals in rural settings.

Specific latitudes and seasons also have an effect. For example, in Boston, USA, located at 42 degrees North, the cutaneous conversion is greatest during June and July. The efficiency of cutaneous conversion declines after August, and by November there is no detectable production of Vitamin D_3 in human skin. Between the months of November and February, exposure to five hours or less of sunlight on cloudless days did not result in any significant production of vitamin D_3. Production resumed in mid-March.[6]

Thus there is no one answer to the question of whether the exclusively breastfed infant should receive vitamin D supplements to prevent development of rickets. The complex relationship between many factors puts, for example, inner city, African American infants in Chicago, or Indian infants in London, at particularly high risk of developing rickets. What is best for the Caucasian infant in Australia may not be best for a Muslim baby in Canada, and the question of whether vitamin D supplements are needed must be answered according to relevant risk factors present for individual infants.

Rickets was a common childhood illness at the turn of the 20th century. In 1898, 80% of children under the age of two in one Boston hospital showed physical signs of rickets. Also known as 'the English disease', rickets was present in epidemic proportions, and not only among infants, in the industrialized cities of northern Europe.[7] By the 1950s and 60s, with vitamin D fortification of infant formula, milk and other foods, the disease became rare. Recently, however, a re-emergence of rickets has been linked with an increase in breastfeeding rates.[8-16]

Bachrach and colleagues published an article in *Pediatrics* of 24 cases of rickets diagnosed at the Children's Hospital in Philadelphia between 1974 and 1978. All infants were breastfed, all were black, and none had received vitamin supplementation. Nineteen of the 24 were members of Muslim or Seventh Day Adventist faiths. Long garments with hoods and veils, and urban pollution, were cited as limiting endogenous synthesis of vitamin D; many of the mothers were vitamin D deficient as well.[17] Another report, out of North Carolina, reviewed records of infants with rickets referred to an endocrinology practice between 1990 and 1999. Thirty cases of rickets were identified; all were African American breastfed infants, and none were on vitamin supplementation. The average age of diagnosis was 12.5 months and most children showed growth retardation (of weight and height) by the time of diagnosis. The authors commented on the increase in breastfeeding rates in North Carolina (WIC data) among all women and African American women during this time period as well.[9]

Food for thought

- Traditionally, young children have been fed cod liver oil to prevent and cure rickets. In 1918, cod liver oil was shown to have antirachitic properties, which were initially ascribed to the vitamin A found in cod liver oil, but even when cod liver oil was heated and exposed to oxygen, thus destroying the vitamin A activity, it retained its antirachitic properties. Since the names Vitamin A, B, and C were already taken, in 1923, the name vitamin D was assigned to the agent in cod liver oil that gave it its antirachitic properties. By 1970, vitamin D was found to be an endogenous steroid precursor, actually a hormone and not a vitamin, but the name remained.

• Vitamin D_2 (ergosterol) becomes biologically active when irradiated.   Until a ready-synthesized form of vitamin D_2 was synthesized, fortified milk was routinely irradiated.[6,7]

References

1. Work Group on Breastfeeding, American Academy of Pediatrics. Breastfeeding and the Use of Human Milk.   *Pediatrics* 1997;100(6):1035-39.
2. Standing Committee on the Scientific Evaluation of Dietary Reference Intakes, Food and Nutrition Board.   *Dietary reference intakes for calcium, phosphorus, magnesuim, vitamin D and fluoride.*   In. Washington, DC: National Academy Press; 1997. p. 250-87.
3. Behrman RE, Kliegman RM, Jenson HB.   *Nelson Textbook of Pediatrics.* 16th ed. Philadelphia: W.B.Saunders Company; 2000.
4. American Academy of Pediatrics, Committee on Nutrition. *Pediatric Nutrition Handbook.*   Elk Grove Village, IL: American Academy of Pediatrics, 1993.
5. American Academy of Pediatrics Committee on Environmental Health. Ultraviolet light: A hazard to children.   *Pediatrics* 1999;104(2):328-333.
6. Holick MF.   McCollum Award Lecture.   Vitamin D: New horizons for the 21st century.   *Am J Clin Nut* 1994;64(6):871-77.
7. Welch TR, Bergstrom WH, Tsang RC.   Vitamin D-deficient rickets: the re-emergence of a once-conquered disease.   *J Pediatr* 2000;137(2):143-5.
8. Eugster EA, Sane KS, Brown DM.   Minnesota rickets.   Need for a policy change to support vitamin D supplementation.   *Minn Med* 1996;79(8):29-32.
9. Kreiter SR, Schwartz RP, Kirkman HN, Jr., Charlton PA, Calikoglu AS, Davenport ML.   Nutritional rickets in African American breast-fed infants.   *J Pediatr* 2000;137(2):153-7.
10. Ozsoylu S. Breast feeding and rickets. *Lancet* 1977;2(8037):560.
11. Gallagher JC, Riggs BL.   Current concepts in nutrition.   Nutrition and bone disease. *N Engl J Med* 1978;298(4):193-5.
12. Hayward I, Stein MT, Gibson MI.   Nutritional rickets in San Diego. *Am J Dis Child* 1987;141(10):1060-2.
13. Kruger DM, Lyne ED, Kleerekoper M.   Vitamin D deficiency rickets. A report on three cases.   *Clin Orthop* 1987(224):277-83.
14. Feldman KW, Marcuse EK, Springer DA.   Nutritional rickets.   *Am Fam Physician* 1990;42(5):1311-8.
15. Gessner BD, deSchweinitz E, Petersen KM, Lewandowski C. Nutritional rickets among breast-fed black and Alaska Native children. *Alaska Med* 1997;39(3):72-4, 87.
16. Pugliese MT, Blumberg DL, Hludzinski J, Kay S.   Nutritional rickets in suburbia. *J Am Coll Nutr* 1998;17(6):637-41.

17. Bachrach S, Fisher J, Parks JS.   An outbreak of vitamin D deficiency rickets in a susceptible population.

Rubella (German Measles)

Summary
A mother with rubella can breastfeed.

Definition/cause
Rubella is an acute, viral, infectious disease, which can be acquired congenitally or postnatally. In congenital rubella, transmission occurs transplacentally, and the disease commonly presents with the triad of low birth weight (intra-uterine growth retardation), cataracts and heart defects.   The timing of the maternal rubella infection during pregnancy determines the likelihood and severity of anomalies.   If infection occurs during the first month, the risk of birth defects is 50% or greater, in the second month the risk falls to 20-30%, and by the third or fourth month the risk drops to 5%.[1] Postnatally acquired disease is transmitted by direct or droplet contact from nasopharyngeal secretions, and manifests as a low-grade fever, rash, and lymphadenopathy.

Signs and symptoms
The most common anomalies seen in infants born with congenital rubella syndrome are ophthalmologic (cataracts, microophthalmia, glaucoma, retinopathy), cardiac (patent ductus arteriosus and stenosis of the pulmonary artery), auditory (sensorineural deafness), and neurologic. Infants may be born with hepatosplenomegaly, "blueberry muffin" rash, and jaundice. Infants born with congenital rubella are usually considered infectious until at least one year of age, and precautions should be taken to prevent their exposure to pregnant women.[1]

Postnatally acquired disease is characterized by low-grade fever, coryza, conjunctivitis, cough, lymphadenopathy (especially involving the suboccipital, post auricular and cervical nodes), and an erythematous maculopapular rash which starts on the face and moves down the trunk to the lower extremities. The illness is self-limiting.

Typically, the virus replicates in the nasopharyngeal mucosa, involves the regional lymph system, and then induces a viremia. An individual with postnatally acquired rubella is most contagious several days before the onset of the rash.

Treatment
Vaccination is the best method of preventing rubella infection. Treatment is symptomatic.

Rubella and breastfeeding
A woman or an infant with rubella can breastfeed. The rubella virus has been isolated from breastmilk both after a maternal infection, and after maternal immunization with the rubella virus vaccine,[2-5] which contains a live attenuated virus. Rubella antibodies have also been found in breastmilk.[6] Some reports suggest that rubella may be transmitted to the infant via breastmilk,[2] however, the rubella virus in breastmilk has not been associated with significant disease in infants, and transmission is more likely to occur via alternate routes.[1] Thus the mother with rubella, or the mother who has been immunized against rubella, can continue to breastfeed.[1,6]

Food for thought
• Attenuated rubella virus vaccine was developed in the 1960s and licensed for use in the USA in 1969.
• Only one type of rubella virus has been described.

References
1. American Academy of Pediatrics. In:Pickering LK. ed. *2000 Red Book: Report of the Committee on Infectious Diseases*. 25th ed. Elk Grove Village, IL:American Academy of Pediatrics; 2000.
2. May JT. Microbial contaminants and antimicrobial properties of human milk. *Microbiol Sci* 1988;5(2):42-6.
3. Losonsky GA, Fishaut JM, Strussenberg J, Ogra PL. Effect of immunization against rubella on lactation products. I. Development and characterization of specific immunologic reactivity in breast milk. *J Infect Dis* 1982;145(5):654-60.
4. Losonsky GA, Fishaut JM, Strussenberg J, Ogra PL. Effect of immunization against rubella on lactation products. II. Maternal-neonatal interactions. *J Infect Dis* 1982;145(5):661-6.

5. Buimovici-Klein E, Hite RL, Byrne T, Cooper LZ. Isolation of rubella virus in milk after postpartum immunization. *J Pediatr* 1977;91(6):939-41.
6. Lawrence RA, Lawrence RM. *Breastfeeding: A Guide for the Medical Profession.* 5th ed. St. Louis: Mosby; 1999:585.

Sheehan's syndrome

Summary

Sheehan's syndrome can cause lactation failure.

Definition/cause

Sheehan's syndrome, which occurs in 0.01% to 0.02% of postpartum women,[1] results from significant postnatal hemorrhage. The hemorrhage leads to systemic hypotension, followed by hypoperfusion, then infarction or necrosis of the pituitary gland. The lateral aspects of the pituitary gland, where most lactotrophs are found, have a precarious blood supply under normal conditions. With pregnancy, hypertrophy of these lactotrophs makes them more sensitive to hypoperfusion and the consequences of infarction and necrosis. Usually, necrosis of the pituitary stalk halts production of prolactin, which leads to lactation failure.[1]

Depending on the degree of damage done to the pituitary gland, the condition can reverse spontaneously.[1]

Signs and symptoms

Signs of Sheehan's syndrome include amenorrhea, diabetes insipidus, hair loss, poor growth of axillary and pubic hair, susceptibility to cold, and lactation failure. Women also usually secrete subnormal levels of pituitary hormones, and have inadequate adrenal and thyroid function.[1] In less severe cases lactation does not fail completely but milk supply may be insufficient. Sheehan's syndrome as a result of postpartum hemorrhage can manifest in the immediate postpartum period, or many years later. One review of six cases found that "the interval between giving birth and the onset of symptoms of hormonal deficiency ranged from three to 32 years."[2]

Sheehan's syndrome and breastfeeding

The hormones prolactin and oxytocin are produced by the pituitary gland and are crucial to successful lactation. Prolactin acts on the mammary glands to synthesize milk, and oxytocin stimulates the myoepithelial cells surrounding mammary alveoli to express milk via the milk ejection reflex. Thus, when the pituitary is damaged, lactation is affected.

Lactation failure is a classic symptom of Sheehan's syndrome. If a mother is not producing enough milk, or if an infant is latching on well to the breast, nursing frequently, but failing to gain weight, Sheehan's syndrome in the mother should be ruled out as a possible cause.

Food for thought

- The longest recorded interval between postpartum hemorrhage and diagnosis of symptoms of Sheehan's syndrome is 48 years. A 68 year old woman with a history prolonged postpartum hemorrhage at age 20 was suffering from severe anemia, weakness, and cold intolerance. In the interim she had resumed menstruation and given birth to two more children, but had a history of poor lactation.[3]

- Hormones secreted by the anterior pituitary include prolactin, growth hormone (GH), thyroid stimulating hormone (TSH), luteinizing hormone (LH), follicle-stimulating hormone (FSH) and adrenocorticotropin hormone (ACTH). Oxytocin and vasopressin (ADH) are hormones secreted by the posterior pituitary.

References

1. Lawrence RA, Lawrence RM. *Breastfeeding: A Guide for the Medical Profession.* 5th ed. St. Louis: Mosby; 1999:513-14.
2. Otsuka F, Kageyama J, Ogura T, Hattori T, Makino H. Sheehan's syndrome of more than 30 years' duration: an endocrine and MRI study of 6 cases. *Endocr J* 1998;45(4):451-8.
3. Ishikawa K, Sohmiya M, Furuya H, Kato Y. A case of Sheehan's syndrome associated with severe anemia and empty sella proved 48 years after postpartum hemorrhage. *Endocr J* 1995;42(6):803-9.

Sickle cell disease (SCD)

Summary

A mother and an infant with sickle cell disease can breastfeed.

Definition/cause

Sickle cell disease is an autosomal recessive genetic disorder, which results in the production of an abnormal hemoglobin, hemoglobin S. The disease is seen in many population groups, but is most common in those of African descent. Approximately 8% of African-Americans are carriers and have sickle cell *trait,* which is benign.

Hemoglobin is a complex protein made up of a heme component, containing iron, and two pairs of globin chain, with each chain containing 150 amino acids. The role of hemoglobin in the body is to transport oxygen reversibly. In sickle hemoglobin (Hb S), valine takes the place normally occupied by glutamic acid at the sixth position of the beta chain. In the oxygenated form, Hb S functions normally, however, when deoxygenated, and under certain stresses, it elongates and causes the red blood cell to take on a sickle shape. The sickled red blood cells have a shortened life span and tend to obstruct small blood vessels, causing tissue hypoxia, ischemia and necrosis.

Signs and symptoms

Adults with sickle cell disease suffer from a chronic hemolytic anemia, with hemoglobin levels ranging from 5-9 g/dL, and from periodic "crises" associated with the condition. Fever, hypoxia, dehydration, and acidosis cause hemoglobin to deoxygenate and may precipitate a crisis, for example, when the patient has an infectious illness; at other times the cause of the crisis is unknown.

The most common crisis, the painful *vasoocclusive crisis,* occurs when sickled cells obstruct small blood vessels causing tissue hypoxia, ischemia and death in bones, joints, the abdomen (this may mimic surgical abdomen), lung (acute chest), and brain (stroke). The other types of crises are *sequestration crisis,* in which large amounts of blood becomes pooled in abdominal organs, especially the spleen, and *aplastic crisis,* which affects the bone marrow.

The destruction of splenic tissue from sickled cells and poor blood flow results in functional asplenia and the inability to destroy encapsulated bacteria. As a result, individuals with SCD are at particular risk of pneumococcal sepsis and salmonella osteomyelitis. In infants, detection is often from mandated state newborn screening results. Otherwise, the disease does not declare itself until after six months of age, when Hb S replaces fetal hemoglobin (Hb F). Often the first sign of illness in an infant with sickle cell disease is acute dactylitis ('hand-foot syndrome'), causing symmetrically swollen and painful hands and feet.

Treatment

The common, repetitive vasoocclusive crises often require hospitalization, intravenous hydration and pain medication, and antibiotics as necessary.

SCD patients are treated prophylactically with penicillin and folic acid, and should be fully immunized. Hydroxyurea is a new treatment that stimulates erythropoiesis, increasing the production of hemoglobin F. Patients may require chronic transfusions; bone marrow transplantation offers a cure.

Sickle cell disease and breastfeeding

Breastfeeding is recommended for the infant diagnosed with sickle cell disease. The mother should be encouraged to follow the American Academy of Pediatrics guidelines[1] and provide breastmilk exclusively for approximately the first six months of life. Breastmilk protects against infection,[2-6] and women should be encouraged to breastfeed these infection-prone babies through the first year of life and beyond wherever possible.

The woman with SCD who wants to breastfeed should be supported in her choice. She will need to pay careful attention to hydration, remaining maximally hydrated at all times, but especially during any sort of crisis. Pain medications such as acetaminophen, codeine, and others used in these situations are usually compatible with breastfeeding.

Food for thought

- The red blood cells of individuals with sickle cell trait resist invasion by the malaria parasite.

Resources

Sickle Cell Disease Association of America
200 Corporate Pointe, Ste. 495
Culver City, CA 90203
Tel. 800/421-8453
Tel. 310/216-6363

Sickle Cell Disease Association of the Piedmont
1102 E. Market St.
Greensboro, NC 27401
Tel. 800/733-8297
Tel. 336/274-1507
www.greensboro.com/sickle/

Sickle Cell Society
6999 Cote des Neiges, Ste. 33
Montreal, PQ CAN H3S 2B8
514/735-5109

References

1. American Academy of Pediatrics Work Group on Breastfeeding. Breastfeeding and the Use of Human Milk. *Pediatrics* 1997;100(6):1035-1039.
2. Beaudry M, Dufour R, Marcoux S. Relation between infant feeding and infections during the first six months of life. *J Pediatr* 1995;126(2):191-7.
3. Dewey KG, Heinig MJ, Nommsen-Rivers LA. Differences in morbidity between breast-fed and formula-fed infants. *J Pediatr* 1995;126(5 Pt 1):696-702.
4. Hanson LA. Human milk and host defence: immediate and long-term effects. *Acta Paediatr Suppl* 1999;88(430):42-6.
5. Howie PW, Forsyth JS, Ogston SA, Clark A, Florey CD. Protective effect of breast feeding against infection. *BMJ* 1990;300(6716):11-6.
6. Victora CG, Smith PG, Vaughan JP, et al. Evidence for protection by breast-feeding against infant deaths from infectious diseases in Brazil. *Lancet* 1987;2(8554):319-22.

Surgery

Summary
Surgery is rarely a contraindication to breastfeeding.

Definition/cause
Surgical operations vary from elective procedures such as gall bladder removal in the mother, or bringing down an undescended testicle in the baby boy, to potentially life-saving procedures such as correcting cardiac anomalies.

Surgery and breastfeeding
Maternal surgery
(See also: Augmentation mammoplasty, Reduction mammoplasty, Breast abscess, Cancer, Galactoceles)

Reasons for surgery differ widely.   On rare occasions, the circumstances surrounding specific maternal surgeries, or the illnesses which lead to surgery, may make weaning necessary. However, many types of surgery present no reason to wean the infant, and breastfeeding can resume as soon as the mother recovers from the anesthesia and is physically capable of nursing the child. Surgery is an upheaval in family life, especially where a young child is involved, and unnecessarily suggesting that the mother wean only adds stress to the situation.

Surgical considerations
Prior to her surgery, the mother should investigate hospital policies regarding rooming-in for infants. Some hospitals (such as Boston Medical Center, Boston) will allow this if a second person is available to stay and care for the infant when the mother is incapacitated, and while the nursing staff cares for the mother. The mother may be able to choose to have the procedure at an institution with a generous policy in this area. If no such policy exists, the mother of an exclusively breastfed young infant may decide to postpone elective surgery until the baby is older and eating other foods. It is worth investigating this policy even if the procedure is only considered day surgery, in case complications cause the mother to remain hospitalized longer than anticipated.

If separation is inevitable, alternate feeding methods should be in place for the young, exclusively breastfeeding infant, because the mother may not be well enough to nurse immediately after surgery, or complications may make her indisposed for longer than anticipated. Similarly, the mother may want to take a high quality breast pump to the hospital (or be sure the hospital has one available for her) to pump milk for the baby, and reduce the chance of engorgement, if the baby is to be separated from her after the operation.

Anesthesia

Often, concern is expressed over anesthesia.   Women may erroneously be advised to 'pump and dump' following general anesthesia, or to postpone elective surgery because anesthesia is best avoided whilst breastfeeding.   In reality, many anesthetic agents are compatible with breastfeeding.

Anesthetic agents are usually used for short periods of time. They remain in the plasma (whence they are transferred into the milk) only briefly, at low levels, before being redistributed to other tissues. As a combined result of these factors, the levels of anesthesia in human milk are generally extremely low, whether the anesthetic is local or general.[1] Some anesthetics have been studied in breastfeeding mothers, and many (including bupivcaine, fentanyl, halothane, ketorolac, lidocaine, lorazepam, morphine, and thiopental sodium) are approved by the American Academy of Pediatrics for use in breastfeeding mothers.   According to Hale, "without exception, the transfer of local anesthetics into human milk is extremely low."[1]

Infant surgery

(See also Cleft lip and palate, Pyloric stenosis)

The mother whose infant needs surgery should be encouraged to continue breastfeeding up until the day of surgery, and to maintain lactation by means of an electric breast pump until the infant is able to return to breast after the operation.   The infection-reducing properties of breastmilk are particularly valuable for a sick infant.[2-5]

The most pertinent question surrounding infant or toddler surgery is the timing of breastfeeds before and after surgery.   Guidelines published by the American Society of Anesthesiologists support a fasting period of four hours from breastmilk, for infants requiring general anesthesia, regional anesthesia, or sedation/analgesia, compared to a six hour fasting period from formula.[6] Some hospitals are less conservative: Children's Hospital in Boston, Massachusetts, considers breastmilk a clear fluid and encourages breastfeeding up to three hours before surgery. Their "Guidelines for Eating and Drinking before Surgery", for infants and young children, state: "You may give clear liquids up to three hours before surgery. Clear liquids include breastmilk, infant electrolyte solution, apple juice, and sugar water." Formula must not be given fewer than six hours before surgery.[7] They then allow the nursing baby to be put to the breast immediately the infant recovers from anesthesia and wants to drink, unless, of course, oral feeds are contraindicated.

References

1. Hale   TW.   *Clinical   Therapy   in Breastfeeding Patients.* Amarillo:Pharmasoft Publishing, 1999:17-23.
2. Beaudry M, Dufour R, Marcoux S.   Relation between infant feeding and infections during the first six months of life. *J Pediatr* 1995;126(2):191-7.
3. Dewey KG, Heinig MJ, Nommsen-Rivers LA.   Differences in morbidity between breast-fed and formula-fed infants.   *J Pediatr* 1995;126(5 Pt 1):696-702.
4. Hanson LA.   Human milk and host defence: immediate and long-term effects. *Acta Paediatr Suppl* 1999;88(430):42-6.
5. Howie PW, Forsyth JS, Ogston SA, Clark A, Florey CD.   Protective effect of breast feeding against infection. *BMJ* 1990;300(6716):11-6.
6. Practice   Guidelines   for   Preoperative   Fasting and the Use of Pharmacologic Agents to Reduce the Risk of Pulmonary Aspiration: Application to Healthy Patients Undergoing Elective Procedures. American Society of Anesthesiologists;Task Force on Preoperative Fasting and the Use of Pharmacologic Agents to Reduce the Risk of Pulmonary Aspiration.
7. Guidelines for Eating and Drinking before Surgery, Family Education and Resource Program, Children's Hospital, 300 Longwood Ave., Boston, MA 02115

Syphilis

Summary
A woman who is diagnosed with syphilis should receive prompt treatment. An infant with signs of syphilis, or at high risk of developing syphilis, should also receive prompt treatment. As long as treatment is initiated or is about to be initiated, a mother or an infant with syphilis can breastfeed. If mother and infant are being treated but are separated, the mother can pump her milk for her child.

Definition/cause
Syphilis is a multisystem infectious disease caused by the spirochete, *Treponema pallidum*. Because the organism does not survive long outside the host, syphilis is not highly contagious; direct inoculation is needed for transmission.

In acquired syphilis, sexual transmission is the most common mode of infection, usually via the genital organs, and contact with infected open skin lesions or mucous membranes. With congenital syphilis, transmission is usually transplacental, occurring at any time during the pregnancy, or by infant contact with spirochetes during passage through the birth canal.

Signs and symptoms
Syphilis progresses in three stages: primary, secondary, and tertiary.

In primary syphilis, the spirochete enters the body through an open area or mucous membrane, multiplies, and disseminates body-wide. Within three to four weeks, an inflammatory response, called a chancre, occurs at the site of the inoculation. A chancre is often found in the genital area, is loaded with spirochetes, and is usually solitary, non-tender and firm. Nearby are enlarged, non-tender lymph nodes. If untreated, the chancre will heal spontaneously leaving only a small scar. If the patient is pregnant during the primary stage, the result is often spontaneous abortion or a stillbirth: perinatal death occurs in 40% of cases.[1]

If the patient remains untreated, the secondary stage begins two to 10 weeks after the chancre heals. The patient will have flu-like symptoms due to spirochetemia; fever, sore throat, a maculopapular rash all over the body with a predilection for the palms and soles, lymphadenopathy, condylomata lata (wart like plaques in moist areas around anus and vagina), and white mucous patches in the mouth. This is followed by a latent period, which may last years, in which the patient is seroactive but there is no other evidence of the disease. In the final stage, tertiary syphilis, any organ system can be affected, and gummata - granulomas of skin and musculoskeletal system due to delayed hypersensitivity reaction - occur. Complications include invasion of the neurological and cardiovascular systems.

Two thirds of infected infants who survive syphilis *in utero* and perinatally are asymptomatic at birth. They are identified by routine newborn screening where available. Early stage manifestations of congenital syphilis are varied and involve many organ systems: characteristic X-ray findings include osteochondritis and periostitis of long bones, particularly the femur and humerus, and rhinitis or 'snuffles' occurring at around one week of age. At approximately three weeks a characteristic rash develops, and simultaneous symptoms may include skin fissures, mucous patches, hemolytic anemia, thrombocytopenia, pneumonia, hepatosplenomegaly, and jaundice. Late stage manifestations result from chronic inflammation of bones, teeth, and the central nervous system.

The organism is difficult to culture, thus diagnosis is made using serology nontreponemal screening tests: both VDRL (Venereal Disease Research Laboratory) and RPR (rapid plasma reagin) detect antibodies against a cardiolipin-cholesterol-lecithin complex (not specific for syphilis). Titers rise with active disease and decline when treatment is adequate. There are also tests that measure antibodies specific for *Treponema pallidum*: TPI, FTA-ABS, MHA-TP, which are usually performed to confirm a positive screening test.

Treatment

Treponema pallidum is extremely sensitive to penicillin. The patient should be screened for other sexually transmitted diseases like gonorrhea, chlamydia, HIV, and hepatitis B, and a history should be obtained for herpes and venereal warts. Any sexual contacts should also be screened and treated. Counseling regarding the dangers of this disease is appropriate. Routine prenatal screening should take place during pregnancy, with more frequent screening for high risk mothers. An infant at high risk of developing the disease needs to be treated. Infants are considered high risk if :[2]

- They are born to a mother with untreated syphilis at delivery
- There is evidence of maternal relapse or reinfection
- They show physical evidence of active disease
- There is radiologic evidence of syphilis
- There is a reactive CSF VDRL, or, for infants born to seropositive mothers, an abnormal CSF white blood cell count or protein, regardless of CSF serology.
- A serum quantitative nontreponemal serologic titer in the infant is at least fourfold greater than the mother's titer.

Syphilis and breastfeeding

A mother and/or a newborn with open lesions should be separated from each other for 24 hours, isolated from other mothers and infants for 24 hours, and both should be started on penicillin therapy.

To date no transmission has been reported of *Treponema pallidum* in breastmilk, however data in this area is lacking. As long as mother and infant are receiving appropriate penicillin therapy, or are about to receive therapy, breastfeeding should begin and continue as usual.

Food for thought

- Syphilis was first recognized in Europe at the end of the 15th century but its sexual transmission was not understood until the 18th century.[1]
- *Treponema pallidum* was discovered in 1905 by Schaudinn and Hoffman.[1]
- The first blood test for the disease was reported in 1906 by Wassermann.[1]
- Syphilis is a fascinating multisystem disease, which lays claim to a varied and unusual terminology including frontal bossing, olympian brow, Higoumenakis sign, saber shins, pseudoparalysis of Parrot, mulberry molars, Hutchinson teeth, saddle nose,

rhagades, Clutton joints, snuffles, eighth cranial nerve deafness, gumma, condylomata lata, and interstitial keratitis.

References

1. Feigin RD, Cherry JD eds. *Textbook of Pediatric Infectious Diseases.* 4th ed. Philadelphia:WB Saunders;1998:1543-1556
2. Centers for Disease Control: 1998 Guidelines for treatment of sexually transmitted diseases. MMWR 47(RR-1):1, 1998
3. Lawrence RA, Lawrence RM. *Breastfeeding: A Guide for the Medical Profession.* 5th ed. St. Louis: Mosby; 1999:606-7.

Toxoplasmosis

Summary

A mother and a baby with toxoplasmosis can breastfeed.

Definition/cause

Toxoplasmosis is a parasitic infection caused by *Toxoplasma gondii.* The cat is the definitive host, and infection in humans often occurs following contact with sources contaminated by feline feces, such as cat litter, soil, and unwashed garden products. Toxoplasmosis can also be contracted by eating undercooked meat.

In the healthy adult human, toxoplasmosis is often an asymptomatic and self-limiting disease. However, pregnant women with primary toxoplasmosis can transmit the parasite transplacentally, and congenital toxoplasmosis is a serious illness. The chance of the fetus becoming infected depends on the timing of maternal primary infection: the risk of transmission is 25% in the first trimester, 54% in the second trimester, and 65% in the third trimester. However, severity of disease varies inversely with time of infection, thus infants infected during the first trimester have more severe disease than those infected in the second and third trimesters.[1] Congenital toxoplasmosis is a leading cause of fetal death.[2]

Signs and symptoms

Infected neonates who survive the pregnancy are often asymptomatic at birth, with complications emerging later.[1] The organism has an affinity for the central nervous system and the retina, thus eye and central nervous system abnormalities are common. Congenital toxoplasmosis can also cause intracranial calcifications, chorioretinitis, hydrocephalus or microcephaly, hepatosplenomegaly, jaundice, seizures, and abnormal cerebrospinal fluid. Sequelae can include mental retardation, seizures, spasticity, palsies, impaired vision, and hearing deficits.

Treatment

Prevention of congenital toxoplasmosis is best achieved by educating all pregnant women: they should avoid contact with possible contaminated sources such as kitty litter; practice good hand washing after working in the garden, wash garden products, and avoid eating raw and undercooked meat. Prenatal screening tests are available, but are expensive, and treating pregnant women is largely ineffective in terms of fetal outcome.[2-5]

Diagnosis is made by testing the neonate for antibodies to toxoplasmosis, and in many US states, toxoplasmosis is included in the routine newborn screening test. The current recommendation is to treat both symptomatic and asymptomatic congenital toxoplasmosis with pyrimethamine and sulfadiazine.[6] One study found an unexpected reduction or resolution of intracranial calcifications in infants with treated, congenital toxoplasmosis during the first year of life.[7]

Most cases of acquired infection do not require treatment.[6]

Toxoplasmosis and breastfeeding

Women and infants with toxoplasmosis can breastfeed. Transmission of toxoplasmosis in breastmilk has not been demonstrated; antibodies to toxoplasmosis have been found in breastmilk, and if acquired postnatally, the infection is benign.[8]

Food for thought

• **TORCHS** is an acronym for a group of severe congenital and perinatal infections: *Toxoplasmosis*, Rubella, Cytomegalovirus, Chickenpox, Herpes simplex virus, Syphylis.

References
1.   Feigin RD, Cherry JD, eds *Textbook of Pediatric Infectious Diseases.*
     4th ed. Philadelphia: WB Saunders; 1998:2473:90.
2.   Derouin F, Jacqz-Aigrain E, Thulliez P, Couvreur J, Leport C.
     Cotrimoxazole for prenatal treatment of congenital toxoplasmosis?
     Parasitol Today 2000;16(6):254-6.
3.   Lebech M, Andersen O, Christensen NC, et al.   Feasibility of neonatal
     screening for toxoplasma infection in the absence of prenatal treatment.
     Danish   Congenital   Toxoplasmosis   Study   Group.   *Lancet*
     1999;353(9167):1834-7.
4.   Peyron F, Wallon M, Liou C, Garner P.   Treatments for toxoplasmosis
     in pregnancy. *Cochrane Database Syst Rev* 2000;2.
5.   Wallon M, Liou C, Garner P, Peyron F.   Congenital toxoplasmosis:
     systematic review of evidence of efficacy of treatment in pregnancy.
     BMJ 1999;318(7197):1511-4.
6.   American Academy of Pediatrics.   In: Pickering LK, ed. *2000 Red
     Book: Report of the Committee on Infectious Diseases.*   25 ed.   Elk
     Grove Village, IL: American Academy of Pediatrics; 2000:583-86.
7.   Patel DV, Holfels EM, Vogel NP, Boyer KM, Mets MB, Swisher CN, et
     al.   Resolution of intracranial calcifications in infants with treated
     congenital toxoplasmosis. *Radiology* 1996;199(2):433-40.
8.   Lawrence RA, Lawrence RM. *Breastfeeding: A Guide for the Medical
     Profession.* 5th ed.   St.   Louis: Mosby, 1999:607-8.

Tracheoesophageal fistula (TE fistula)

Summary
The infant with TE fistula may not be able to eat by mouth
for some time while the anomaly is surgically corrected.   The
mother should be encouraged and supported to maintain her
milk supply by pumping during this time, with the greater goal of
direct breastfeeding when surgical repair of the esophagus is
complete and healed.

Definition/cause
Esophageal atresia with or without TE fistula is the most common
anomaly of the esophagus, occurring in between 1:2000 and 1:5000
live births.[1]   Five forms of esophageal atresia with TE fistula can
occur, the most common, which accounts for approximately 85% of

cases, involves a proximal esophageal pouch and a fistula connecting the trachea to the distal esophagus.[1]

Signs and symptoms

The newborn with a TE fistula will present with copious oral secretions, respiratory distress, and possible aspiration. Failure to pass a nasogastric tube is diagnostic, and the condition can be confirmed by an x-ray which will reveal the tube coiled in the pouch. In 50% of cases, maternal polyhydramnios is present.

Treatment

The aim of treatment is to identify and tie off the fistula and reconnect the esophagus. Primary anastomosis of the esophagus is the ideal, however this may not be possible, in which case chronic elongation, and use of the colon, the stomach, or tissue from other areas of the body may be necessary. If the infant is healthy, surgery is usually performed as soon after diagnosis as possible. However, the infant may have initial complications from failed feeds or aspirated milk, which may need to be resolved. During the recovery phase, the infant is maintained in a position with the head elevated.

TE fistula and breastfeeding

The mother of an infant with TE fistula should be encouraged to provide breastmilk for a baby who will undergo surgery and remain hospitalized for a considerable time. Breastmilk lowers the risk of infection,[2-6] and, as an easily digested fluid, is the best possible form of nutrition for a baby with a susceptible digestive tract.[7] However, the mother will need a great deal of encouragement around pumping in the early stages, because her milk may not be fed to her infant for some time. Some milk may be given in the early post-operative period if the baby is being fed through a gastronomy tube,[7] otherwise the infant may start to breastfeed when the surgery is healed and the baby is ready to begin oral feeds (see Surgery).

The clinician should encourage the mother to obtain a high quality electric breast pump as soon as possible after birth, and to pump her breasts approximately every three hours for 10-15 minutes in order to create and maintain a milk supply throughout the period when the baby cannot nurse (see Breastfeeding aids). She should be reassured that all milk will be frozen and given to the hospitalized baby during the recovery period if the mother is not available to breastfeed.

Food for thought

- This condition is one of a series of related anomalies which are described with the acronym VACTERL. The acronym stands for: Vertebral Anomalies, Cardiac defects, **TE** fistula, **R**enal or **R**adial anomalies, and **L**imb malformations.

Resources

TEF/VATER International Support Network
C/O Greg and Terry Burke
15301 Grey Fox Rd.
Upper Marlboro, MD 20772
Tel. 301/952-6837

References

1. McMillan JA, DeAngelis DC, Feigin RD, Warshaw JB, eds. *Oski's Pediatrics: Principles and Practice.* 3rd ed. Philadelphia: Lippincott Williams and Wilkins; 1999:309-311.
2. Beaudry M, Dufour R, Marcoux S. Relation between infant feeding and infections during the first six months of life. *J Pediatr* 1995;126(2):191-7.
3. Dewey KG, Heinig MJ, Nommsen-Rivers LA. Differences in morbidity between breast-fed and formula-fed infants. *J Pediatr* 1995;126(5 Pt 1):696-702.
4. Hanson LA. Human milk and host defense: immediate and long-term effects. *Acta Paediatr Suppl* 1999;88(430):42-6.
5. Howie PW, Forsyth JS, Ogston SA, Clark A, Florey CD. Protective effect of breast feeding against infection. *BMJ* 1990;300(6716):11-6.
6. Victora CG, Smith PG, Vaughan JP, Nobre LC, Lombardi C, Teixeira AM, et al. Evidence for protection by breast-feeding against infant deaths from infectious diseases in Brazil. *Lancet* 1987;2(8554):319-22.
7. Lawrence RA, Lawrence RM. *Breastfeeding: A Guide for the Medical Profession.* 5th ed. St. Louis: Mosby; 1999:492-93.

Tracheostomy

Summary

If the infant is physically capable of suckling, breastfeeding can continue despite the presence of a tracheostomy.

Definition/cause

A tracheostomy is a tube, placed into the trachea, with an opening (stoma) at the throat, through which an infant with a compromised or otherwise obstructed airway can breathe. Tracheostomies may also be used in infants who have trouble breathing due to neuromuscular diseases involving respiratory compromise, as a sequelae of prematurity, and in tracheomalacia, a newborn condition where the trachea collapses at the end of each breath.

The infant with a tracheostomy breathes through the stoma at the throat.   This opening must be kept clear and unblocked at all times or the child risks suffocation. Air entering the stoma should be kept moist, to prevent secretions from drying out and blocking the tracheostomy. Methods of keeping air and secretions moist include a specially designed humidifier, with a hose and mask device, which can be fitted loosely around the infant's neck over the stoma. An 'artificial nose' – a cylinder which fits snugly over the open end of the tracheostomy, containing a paper filter – also keeps the air and airway moist. The tracheostomy tube should be suctioned regularly to keep it clear.

Tracheostomy and breastfeeding

Unless the infant with a tracheostomy has other complicating factors (such as neurological problems which impair the suck swallow mechanism), breastfeeding can continue in the presence of the tracheostomy. Breastfeeding is recommended for these compromised babies because it lowers the risk of infection in general,[1-5] and the risk of respiratory tract infection in particular.[3-11] If the infant is physically unable to nurse, the mother should be encouraged to provide breastmilk for her child by using an electric breast pump (see Prematurity for details on pumping for sick infants).

The infant will need initial surgery to fit the tracheostomy, and will probably need future surgery to remove it and/or to repair a damaged airway. If possible, nursing should begin in the newborn period, before the surgery. The mother will then need to pump throughout the surgical and recovery periods to maintain her milk supply, and to provide milk which can be fed to the baby by alternate means until the s/he is able to nurse.

The nursing mother will need to take extra care with positioning, in order to ensure that nothing (such as her clothing) obstructs the entry to the tracheostomy. The cradle hold may work better than the football hold for these infants, because the throat is obscured from the mother when using the football hold. Spit up must not enter the tracheostomy because it will choke the baby, and some mothers may feel more comfortable nursing with the artificial nose in place to prevent this. The mother may decide to breastfeed with the humidifier and mask in place, especially if she is nursing the infant to sleep, and plans to leave the mask in place during the nap. As the baby grows and becomes more mobile, the parents may find themselves using the artificial nose more frequently, as it is less cumbersome than the humidifier, hose, and mask combination.

As with any chronically sick infant, breastfeeding normalizes the experience for the mother.

Food for thought

• Isabel breathed through a tracheostomy from day four of life until 10 months of age, when surgery successfully repaired a laryngeal web and her narrow airway. Her mother recalls, "Of course, breastfeeding is best because of all the health benefits for the baby. But for the mother's mental health it is invaluable. Doctors are always whisking the baby away, and even though they are saving her life, you hate all the intervention, it goes against every maternal instinct. Breastfeeding was the one thing I could do that none of the doctors could do. It was the only contribution I could make. Everything else was out of my hands."

References
1. Beaudry M, Dufour R, Marcoux S. Relation between infant feeding and infections during the first six months of life. *J Pediatr* 1995;126(2):191-7.

2. Dewey KG, Heinig MJ, Nommsen-Rivers LA.   Differences in morbidity between breast-fed and formula-fed infants.   *J Pediatr* 1995;126(5 Pt 1):696-702.
3. Hanson LA.   Human milk and host defense: immediate and long-term effects.   *Acta Paediatr Suppl* 1999;88(430):42-6.
4. Howie PW, Forsyth JS, Ogston SA, Clark A, Florey CD.   Protective effect of breast feeding against infection.   *BMJ* 1990;300(6716):11-6.
5. Victora CG, Smith PG, Vaughan JP, Nobre LC, Lombardi C, Teixeira AM, et al.   Evidence for protection by breast-feeding against infant deaths from infectious diseases in Brazil.   *Lancet* 1987;2(8554):319-22.
6. Forman MR, Graubard BI, Hoffman HJ, Beren R, Harley EE, Bennett P.   The Pima infant feeding study: breastfeeding and respiratory infections during the first year of life.   *Int J Epidemiol* 1984;13(4):447-53.
7. Burr ML, Limb ES, Maguire MJ, Amarah L, Eldridge BA, Layzell JC, et al.   Infant feeding, wheezing, and allergy: a prospective study.   *Arch Dis Child* 1993;68(6):724-8.
8. Ford K, Labbok M.   Breast-feeding and child health in the United States.   *J Biosoc Sci* 1993;25(2):187-94.
9. Golding J, Emmett PM, Rogers IS.   Does breast feeding protect against non-gastric infections?   *Early Hum Dev* 1997;49 Suppl:S105-20.
10. Victora CG, Smith PG, Barros FC, Vaughan JP, Fuchs SC.   Risk factors for deaths due to respiratory infections among Brazilian infants.   *Int J Epidemiol* 1989;18(4):918-25.
11. Victora CG, Kirkwood BR, Ashworth A, Black RE, Rogers S, Sazawal S, et al.   Potential interventions for the prevention of childhood pneumonia in developing countries: improving nutrition.   *Am J Clin Nutr* 1999;70(3):309-20.

Trichomoniasis (Trichomonas infection)

Summary

A mother with trichomoniasis can breastfeed, but may need to 'pump and dump' for a short period following metronidazole single dose therapy.

Definition/cause

Trichomonas vaginalis, a pear-shaped, motile protozoal parasite, is a pathogen of the human genitourinary tract. Trichomoniasis, or infection with *Trichomonas vaginalis*, is a venereal disease which causes vaginitis in females, although some women and most males may be asymptomatic. The disease is typically detected among persons with multiple sexual partners and in those with other sexually transmitted diseases (STDs).

Signs and symptoms

Trichomonas vaginalis causes vaginitis with foul smelling, frothy, yellow vaginal discharge and vulvovaginal erythema, itching and/or dysuria. Diagnosis is often made by detecting motile trichomanonads in a wet mount preparation of the vaginal discharge. Culture and antibody testing are other modes of detection. Trichomonas can also be reported coincidentally from urine samples or Pap smears.

Treatment

The single most effective treatment, with a cure rate of 95%,[1] is metronidazole (Flagyl); a one-time, 2 gm oral dose is recommended for adolescents and adults.[1] Sexual partners should be treated at the same time, even if asymptomatic, and the patient and sexual partners should screened for other STDs.

Trichomoniasis medications and breastfeeding

Metronidazole is an antibiotic, used for anaerobic bacterial infections, and an amebicide, used as the treatment of choice for pediatric giardiasis. Currently its use in nursing mothers is controversial. Metronidazole is listed by the American Academy of Pediatrics (AAP) as a 'drug whose effect on nursing infants is unknown but may be of concern'.[2] The present recommendation for a nursing mother taking a one-time, 2 gm oral dose of metronidazole is to pump and dump her milk for '12-24' hours,[3-5] after which breastfeeding can resume. Twelve hours after taking the 2 gm dose, maternal plasma levels are at approximately 20% of the peak blood level, which occurs around two hours after administration.[3]

According to the *Physician's Desk Reference* (PDR), "because of the potential for tumorigenicity shown for metronidazole in mouse and rat studies, a decision should be made whether to discontinue nursing or to discontinue the drug, taking into account the importance of the drug for the mother. Metronidazole is secreted into human milk in concentrations similar to those found in plasma."[6] The PDR also notes: "Safety and effectiveness in pediatric patients has not been established, except in the treatment of amebiasis."[6]

Some sources however lean towards advocacy for the use of metronidazole in breastfeeding mothers. In his article *Can we use metronidazole during pregnancy and breastfeeding? Putting an end to the controversy*,[7] Einarson claims, "Recent evidence has shown…,that this drug is not associated with adverse effects during either pregnancy or breastfeeding."[7]   Hale states that "Metronidazole transfer into human milk is moderate to low", and believes that the debate over contraindication "is largely unfounded".[3]   Studies on varied doses of metronidazole have found relatively low amounts transferred via breastmilk to the nursing infant, and no side effects have been reported in breastfeeding infants. One study concluded that the drug can be administered at doses of 400 mg three times a day to women wishing to breastfeed their infants.[8]   In addition, the drug is used in pediatric patients, at a published dose of 10-20 mg per day.[3]

Trichomoniasis and breastfeeding

Women with trichomoniasis can breastfeed.   The issue, as discussed above, is whether nursing mothers on metronidazole can breastfeed.

Food for thought

• The "strawberry cervix" sometimes seen with trichomoniasis is named for its friable, inflamed appearance.[1]
• While metronidazole proved carcinegous in mice and rats studies, it did not cause tumor growth in hamsters.[6]

References

1.   American Academy of Pediatrics.   In: Pickering LK, ed.   *2000 Red Book: Report of the Committee on Infectious Diseases*.   25th ed.   Elk Grove Village, IL: American Academy of Pediatrics; 2000: 588-89.
2.   American Academy of Pediatrics, Committee on Drugs.   The transfer of drugs and other chemicals into human milk.   *Pediatrics* 1994;93:137-150.
3.   Hale TW. *Clinical Therapy in Breastfeeding Patients*.   Amarillo: Pharmasoft Publishing; 1999.
4.   Hale TW. *Medications and Mothers' Milk*.   Amarillo: Pharmasoft Publishing; 2000.

5.   Lawrence RA, Lawrence RM. *Breastfeeding: A Guide for the Medical Profession.* 5th ed. St Louis:Mosby;1999:780-781.
6.   *Physician's Desk Reference.* 54th ed. New Jersey: Medical Economics; 2000:2918.
7.   Einarson A, Ho E, Koren G.   Can we use metronidazole during pregnancy and breastfeeding? Putting an end to the controversy. *Can Fam Physician* 2000;46:1053-4.
8.   Passmore CM, McElnay JC, Rainey EA, D'Arcy PF. Metronidazole excretion in human milk and its effect on the suckling neonate. *Br J Clin Pharmacol* 1988;26(1):45-51.

Tuberculosis (TB)

Summary

Women with a history of a positive tuberculin skin test but no evidence of active disease can breastfeed. Children born to women with active, untreated tuberculosis disease are at risk of contracting the disease through the respiratory route but not through breastmilk. The mother can pump her milk to be fed to the infant until she is considered non-contagious; then the infant can breastfeed directly.[1]

Definition/cause

Tuberculosis (TB) accounts for over 3,000,000 deaths annually, making it the leading infectious cause of death worldwide. In individuals over five years of age, TB causes more deaths than AIDS, malaria, diarrhea, leprosy, and all other tropical diseases combined.[2] Moreover, the incidence of TB is rising dramatically, due in part to the prevalence of HIV/AIDS, and to the development of drug resistant TB strains. Currently 8-10% of tuberculosis cases worldwide are linked to HIV/AIDS infection, but in African nations this association is higher, at 20% or more.[2]

TB is a multisystemic, chronic granulomatous disease caused by *Mycobacterium tuberculosis.* *Mycobacterium tuberculosis* is transmitted from person to person by airborne respiratory droplets when an infected person coughs or sneezes. The tubercle bacilli enter the body via the lung and multiply within the alveoli. Usually the body can mount an effective immune response to tuberculous infection; in the absence of HIV infection or other cause of immunosuppression, only about 10% of infections develop into disease.[2] An individual with tuberculosis *infection* is asymptomatic and can only be identified by a positive tuberculin skin test reaction.[3] An individual with active tuberculosis *disease* goes on to develop symptoms, and can be diagnosed via a positive skin test plus a positive chest X ray, sputum microscopy, and/or evidence of other organ involvement.

Signs and symptoms

In the approximately 10% of infected individuals who develop tuberculosis disease, tuberculosis pulmonary infection may manifest as cough, wheeze, low grade fever, weight loss, night sweats, and malaise. A chest X ray may reveal an infiltrate, hilar adenopathy or pleural effusion (often unilateral). Extra-pulmonary manifestations include cardiac and pericardial tuberculosis (pericarditis), lymphadenopathy, erythema nodosum, meningitis, brain abscess, skeletal tuberculosis (thoracic or lumbar spinal pain), and renal tuberculosis (painless hematuria).

Treatment

Multi-drug resistant strains of *Mycobacterium tuberculosis* are increasing, making treatment challenging.[4] For tuberculous disease, multi-drug therapy is the standard; different regimens include isoniazid (INH), rifampin, pyrazinamide, ethambutol, and/or streptomycin. According to one source, the standard for TB therapy should be: "Treat with multiple drugs in adequate dosages on a regular basis for sufficient duration with expert monitoring."[4]

Tuberculosis medications and breastfeeding

A thorough review of TB medications and breastfeeding is presented in Hale's *Clinical Therapy in Breastfeeding Patients*.[5] Isoniazid, rifampin, ethambutol and streptomycin are all approved by the American Academy of Pediatrics (AAP) for use in breastfeeding women. Pyrazinamide has not been reviewed but milk levels are believed to remain low. Most of these drugs pass into breastmilk but levels transmitted are less than 20% of the therapeutic pediatric dose.[5]

Tuberculosis and breastfeeding

A woman with a history of tuberculous infection (a positive skin test but a negative chest x-ray) may breastfeed.[6]

A woman with untreated, active disease should be separated from her infant until the mother and infant have received appropriate treatment and the danger of infection is past.[7] During this period the mother can pump and her milk can be fed to the infant, because transmission is by respiratory route and not by breastmilk. Once the mother is considered non-contagious, she can breastfeed directly.

There is no contraindication to tuberculin skin testing during pregnancy or while breastfeeding. Also, there is no altered response to the skin test during either period.

Food for thought

- Rifampin turns secretions such as tears, sweat, urine, and breastmilk orange.
- The AAP recommends tuberculosis skin testing be performed in "high-risk groups." A study of 31,926 children receiving well-child care in California determined the following five questions, which accurately identify high risk groups.[8] A yes to all five questions had a 19.4% prevalence of a positive skin test result.

High Risk Evaluation

- **Has your child ever received BCG?**
- **Has there ever been TB or a positive skin test for TB in any household member (including your child, extended family, overnight guests, frequent visitors, babysitters, and daycare providers)?**
- **Was your child born outside the United States?**
- **Has your child lived outside the United States for more than a month?**
- **How would you describe your child's race or ethnicity? (Asian and Hispanic nationality predicted high risk).**

References
1. Lawrence RA, Howard CR. Given the benefits of breastfeeding, are there any contraindications? *Clin Perinatol* 1999;26(2):479-90, viii.
2. Zumla A, Grange J. Tuberculosis. *BMJ* 1998;316:1962-64.
3. Brandli O. The clinical presentation of tuberculosis. *Respiration* 1998;65:97-105.
4. Albino JA, Reichman LB. The treatment of tuberculosis. *Respiration* 1998;1998(65):237-55.
5. Hale TW. *Clinical Therapy in Breastfeeding Patients.* Amarillo: Pharmasoft Publishing, 1999:105.
6. Snider DE, Jr., Powell KE. Should women taking antituberculosis drugs breast-feed? *Arch Intern Med* 1984;144(3):589-90.
7. AAP. *Red Book: Report of the Committee on Infectious Diseases.* 25 ed. Elk Grove Village, IL, 2000.
8. Froehlich H. Presented at international conference sponsored by CDC, *Pediatric News* November 2000 p 18.

Ulcerative colitis

Summary
A mother with ulcerative colitis can breastfeed. Several studies suggest that lack of breastfeeding in the infant is a risk factor for developing ulcerative colitis later in life. Parents with a family history of the disease should be strongly encouraged to breastfeed their child.

Definition/cause
Ulcerative colitis (UC) is a chronic inflammatory bowel disease (IBD), which is believed to result from a combination of genetic and environmental factors.[1,2] The incidence is 15 per 100,000, and is highest in whites, especially in Jews, Europeans, and Northern Americans. Ulcerative colitis is equally prevalent in males and females, and peaks in the second and third decades of life, and again in the fifth and sixth decades.

Unlike Crohn's disease, ulcerative colitis is localized to the colon and rectum, sparing the upper GI tract, is limited to the mucosa, and affects the gut continuously. Nonetheless the two diseases can be confused, and approximately 15% of cases of noninfectious chronic inflammatory colitis cannot be definitively categorized as either Crohn's disease or ulcerative colitis.

Lack of breastfeeding is a risk factor for developing UC.[3-5] Nicotine use is also related to IBD: while smoking cigarettes appears to be associated with the development of Crohn's disease, and to worsen its course (see Crohn's disease), smoking appears to protect against developing UC, and may improve symptoms.[6-8] Recent trials using nicotine therapy have had some beneficial effects for UC patients.[8]

Signs and symptoms

The disease usually begins in the rectum and spreads proximally. Symptoms are chronic, and marked by flares without apparent explanation. Patients often present with bloody and mucous-filled diarrhea; extraintestinal manifestations include pyoderma gangrenosum, sclerosing cholangitis, chronic active hepatitis, ankylosing spondylitis, anemia and hypoalbuminemia. Severe disease can lead to growth failure. The most serious complication, toxic megacolon, occurs in fewer than 5% of patients.

Diagnosis is made by suggestive history, physical exam, radiographic findings, and exclusion of other causes.

Treatment

Total proctocolectomy (removal of the colon) is curative, but this major surgery leaves the patient with an ileostomy. Before such a step is taken, medical management aims to control symptoms and prevent relapses. Rest and a low-residue diet can be combined with sulfasalazine and oral corticosteroid therapy, depending on severity of disease. Sulfasalazine is converted in the colon to 5 aminosalicylic acid and sulfapyridine. Prednisone is frequently used, both orally and rectally.[9]

Ulcerative colitis medications and breastfeeding

A thorough review of treatment options and their significance for breastfeeding women is presented in Hale's *Clinical Therapy in Breastfeeding Patients*.[9] According to the American Academy of Pediatrics (AAP), sulfasalazine can be used with caution in breastfeeding women. Bioavailability is low, as are published levels in milk.[9] Prednisone is approved by the AAP for use in breastfeeding women, and its transfer into milk appears to be low, although the infant's growth should be carefully monitored.[9]

Ulcerative colitis and breastfeeding

Breastfeeding is associated with a reduced risk of developing ulcerative colitis in later life;[3] the mother with ulcerative colitis or with a family history of ulcerative colitis should be encouraged to breastfeed.

Food for thought

* In Hungary, the Roma (Gypsies) have a considerably lower prevalence of UC than the average population.[2]
* IBD sufferers have an above average incidence of multiple sclerosis. One study found the prevalence of MS among IBD patients to be 3.7 times above the MS rate in the general population.[10]
* Subclinical hearing loss has also been associated with ulcerative colitis.[11]

Resources

CCFA: Crohn's and Colitis Foundation of America
386 Park Ave., S 17th Fl.
New York NY 10016
800/932-2423
212/685-3440
www.ccfa.org

Pediatric Crohn's & Colitis Foundation
PO Box 188
Newton MA 02168
617/489-5854

References
1. Cho J.   Update on Inflammatory Bowel Disease Genetics. *Curr Gastroenterol Rep* 2000;2(6):434-439.
2. Karlinger K, Gyorke T, Mako E, Mester A, Tarjan Z.   The epidemiology and the pathogenesis of inflammatory bowel disease. *Eur J Radiol* 2000;35(3):154-67.

3. Rigas A, Rigas B, Glassman M, Yen YY, Lan SJ, Petridou E, et al. Breast-feeding and maternal smoking in the etiology of Crohn's disease and ulcerative colitis in childhood. *Ann Epidemiol* 1993;3(4):387-92.
4. Corrao G, Tragnone A, Caprilli R, Trallori G, Papi C, Andreoli A, et al. Risk of inflammatory bowel disease attributable to smoking, oral contraception and breastfeeding in Italy: a nationwide case-control study. Cooperative Investigators of the Italian Group for the Study of the Colon and the Rectum (GISC). *Int J Epidemiol* 1998;27(3):397-404.
5. Meeuwisse GW. Immunological considerations on breast vs. formula feeding. *Klin Padiatr* 1985;197(4):322-5.
6. Rubin DT, Hanauer SB. Smoking and inflammatory bowel disease. *Eur J Gastroenterol Hepatol* 2000;12(8):855-62.
7. Kozlova I, Dragomir A, Vanthanouvong V, Roomans GM. Effects of nicotine on intestinal epithelial cells in vivo and in vitro: an X-ray microanalytical study. *J Submicrosc Cytol Pathol* 2000;32(1):97-102.
8. Thomas GA, Rhodes J, Green JT, Richardson C. Role of smoking in inflammatory bowel disease: implications for therapy. *Postgrad Med J* 2000;76(895):273-9.
9. Hale TW. *Clinical Therapy in Breastfeeding Patients.* Amarillo: Pharmasoft Publishing; 1999:110.
10. Kimura K, Hunter SF, Thollander MS, Loftus EV, Jr., Melton LJ, 3rd, O'Brien PC, et al. Concurrence of inflammatory bowel disease and multiple sclerosis. *Mayo Clin Proc* 2000;75(8):802-6.
11. Kumar BN, Smith MS, Walsh RM, Green JR. Sensorineural hearing loss in ulcerative colitis. *Clin Otolaryngol* 2000;25(2):143-5.

Unilateral breastfeeding (One-sided nursing)

Summary
Breastfeeding can succeed even if the infant nurses only on one breast.

Definition/cause
Sometimes the cause of one-sided breastfeeding is clear: a flat or inverted nipple makes nursing difficult on one breast, so the newborn opts for the other. Another reason for neonate preference could be a birth injury such as a fractured clavicle, which causes pain when the infant is placed on one side to nurse. In an older infant, similar causes, such as pain from an ear infection, should be ruled out if the

child suddenly refuses one breast.   Frequently, however, babies whimsically pick a favorite breast for no apparent reason.

Signs and symptoms

In this situation, the baby nurses more on one breast than on the other. If the preference persists, eventually, the mother too will show 'signs' of unilateral breastfeeding: the rejected breast will produce less milk and will shrink, while the preferred breast will respond to the extra stimulation by producing more milk, and will enlarge.

One sided nursing and breastfeeding

Some infants show a preference for nursing on a particular breast. In most cases this is a temporary situation of minor significance. Although mothers understandably become concerned about one-sided nursing, one breast can provide adequate nutrition for a baby, and this is rarely a serious or long term problem.

Solutions usually revolve around 'tricking' the baby into taking the unwanted breast, either by feeding on that side when the infant is sleepy, or by nursing the baby in the cradle hold, then sliding the infant surreptitiously onto the other side whilst maintaining exactly the same position.

If the problem is caused by a flat or inverted nipple, and the newborn is latching well on the unaffected side, the mother should both nurse on the 'chosen' side, and continue to offer the rejected breast. Perhaps in their enthusiasm to succeed at breastfeeding, many new mothers waste valuable energy trying to persuade the infant to nurse on the more difficult side. In reality, both mom and baby would be better off taking the easy option for early feeds, whilst optimistically but casually continuing to offer the rejected breast. A breast pump can be useful to pull out a flat or inverted nipple, and to create or maintain a milk supply when the baby is not stimulating one breast.

Breast preference in an older baby may be connected to nipple size or shape, to the speed of the milk flow or letdown reflex, or even to the taste of the milk.(The sodium content of milk rises as a baby weans, and milk in a rarely used breast may well taste different from milk in the other breast).

Food for thought

- The Tanka (boat people) who live on the coastal waters and the rivers of southern China traditionally nurse only on the right breast.[1]
- In rare cases, sudden refusal to nurse on one breast has been linked with breast cancer.[2,3] (See Cancer).

References

1. Ing R, Petrakis NL, Ho JH.   Unilateral breast-feeding and breast cancer. *Lancet* 1977;2(8029):124-7.
2. Saber A, Dardik H, Ibrahim IM, Wolodiger F.   The milk rejection sign: a natural tumor marker. *Am Surg* 1996;62(12):998-9.
3. Goldsmith HS.   Milk-rejection sign of breast cancer.   *Am J Surg* 1974;127(3):280-1.

Upper respiratory tract infection (Common cold)

Summary

Breastfeeding should continue unrestricted when either mother or infant is affected by an upper respiratory tract infection.

Definition/cause

More than 200 viruses can cause upper respiratory tract infections (URIs).   One third of colds are due to rhinoviruses; other common culprits are parainfluenza, RSV, and coronavirus.[1] Colds occur most frequently in fall and winter, and the mode of transmission is respiratory droplets spread by sneezing, coughing, and poor hygiene.

In children, colds are associated with daycare attendance, parental smoking, low socioeconomic status, and crowding.[2]

Signs and symptoms

The common cold is a self-limited illness that usually lasts from seven to ten days, with the worst symptoms occurring in the first few days.

The infant with a URI may be cranky, congested, and either afebrile or have a low grade fever.   Symptoms can include nasal stuffiness, sneezing, coughing, scratchy throat, poor appetite, loose stools, and general malaise. Colds can be associated with ear infections, sinusitis, bronchitis, pneumonia, and asthma. If the symptoms worsen after a week or the infant develops a significant fever, the mother should contact her clinician.

Treatment
Treatment for the infant consists of rest, keeping the child well hydrated, and using methods to clear the nose such as bulb suction, moist air, saline nose drops, and elevation of the head when in a horizontal position. The parents should avoid exposing the infant to tobacco smoke. The clinician may suggest antipyretic medication or oral decongestants as symptomatic relief. Aspirin should be avoided in children under 18 years because of the association with Reye's syndrome.

Upper respiratory tract infections and breastfeeding
Breastfeeding should be encouraged and continue throughout colds, whether the mother or the infant is affected. When the mother has a URI, she will make antibodies to the cold, which will pass into her milk and help to protect the infant. Several studies show that breastfeeding offers protection to infants against URIs.[3-5]

The nursing infant may pull off the breast frequently, because breathing through a congested nose is difficult. In a very young infant the mother might gently suction the nostrils before a feed so that the baby can breathe through the nose while nursing. Feeding in a more upright position may also help.

Food for thought
- "There is just one way to treat a cold and that is with contempt." (Osler)[2]

References
1. Feigin RD, Cherry, JD eds. *Textbook of Pediatric Infectious Diseases.* 4th ed. Philadelphia: Saunders, 1998:128.
2. Szilagy PG. What can we do about the common cold? *Cont Peds.* 1990;7:23-49.
3. Beaudry M, Dufour R, Marcoux S: Relationship between infant feeding and infections during the first six months of life. *J Pediatr.* 1995;126:191.

4. Lopez-Alarcon M, Villalpando S, Fajardo A: Breastfeeding lowers the frequency and duration of acute respiratory infection and diarrhea in infants under six months of age. *J Nutr.* 1997;127:436.
5. Brown KH, Black RE, Lopez de Romana G, et al. Infant-feeding practices and their relationship with diarrheal and other diseases in Huascar (Lima), Peru. *Pediatrics* 1989;**83**(1):31-40.

Urinary tract infection (UTI)

Summary
A mother with a urinary tract infection can breastfeed.

Definition/cause
Normally, urine is a sterile body fluid. A urinary tract infection (UTI) occurs when pathologic microorganisms - usually bacteria, but occasionally viruses - invade the urinary tract and multiply in the urine causing an infection. Women are particularly prone to UTIs because the short urethra and the accessibility of the urethra to vaginal and rectal organisms predispose women to an ascending infection. There is also an association with sexual activity, pregnancy, and vesicoureteral reflux.

A urinary tract infection is defined by anatomic location: in women, lower tract infections, associated primarily with the bladder, are urethritis, cystitis; upper tract infections are associated with the kidney and include pyelonephritis, and renal abscess.

Most UTI infections are monomicrobial, and *Escherichia coli,* a gram negative bacteria, is the cause in 80% of bacterial cases. Chronic or recurrent infections are due to other organisms, again frequently gram negative bacteria, like *Klebsiella, Enterobacter, Proteus,* and *Enterococcus.*

Signs and symptoms
The classic triad of symptoms for bacterial cystitis is dysuria, urgency, and frequency, occasionally accompanied by lower abdominal pain, low grade temperature, and hematuria.

A culture of over 10^5 bacterial colonies per cubic centimeter from a midstream, clean catch voided urine sample, or any bacteria in urine collected by catheter, indicate an infection. Infection is also suspected if urine dip stick (specifically, nitrite test and leukocyte esterase test) and gram stain of the urine are positive. Definitive diagnosis is made by culture of the urine, and treatment is determined by the antibiotic sensitivity of the organism. Because culture results can take one to two days, the patient is often started on an antibiotic first to treat a suspected infection.

Treatment
UTI medications and breastfeeding

For uncomplicated UTIs in breastfeeding mothers, a common therapy is trimethoprim/sulfamethoxazole double strength (160/800 mg) twice daily for three days.[1] Amoxicillin is also used. Both amoxicillin and trimethoprim are approved by the American Academy of Pediatrics (AAP) for use in breastfeeding women. However, because of the possibility of jaundice, sulfonamides should not be used by women who are nursing premies, newborns, or infants under one month of age. UTI therapy in breastfeeding women is discussed at length in Hale's *Clinical Therapy in Breastfeeding Patients*.[1]

The nursing mother with a UTI should drink plenty of fluids.

UTIs and breastfeeding

The infection will not be transmitted through breastmilk. The mother should continue breastfeeding, and her antibiotic therapy should be prescribed with this objective. An infant with a UTI can also continue to breastfeed.

Protective Effects

In a case-control study of the relationship between UTIs in the first six months of life and infant-feeding methods, Pisacane concluded that breastfeeding was protective against the development of UTIs in infants.[2] The study compared 128 case infants with a UTI, aged from birth to six months, with 128 control infants admitted to the same ward with an acute illness. Only 64 (50%) of the infants with UTIs had 'ever been breastfed' compared to 93 (73%) of the control infants (p<0.001)(RR 0.38). Just 16 (12%) of the case infants were "being breastfed" during hospitalization compared to 56 (44%) of the control infants (p<0.001)(RR 0.18).[2]

References

1. Hale TW.   *Clinical Therapy in Breastfeeding Patients.*   Amarillo: Pharmasoft Publishing;1999:176-77.
2. Pisacane A, Graziano L, Mazzarella G, Scarpellino B, Zona G.   Breastfeeding and urinary tract infection.   *J Pediatr* 1992;120(1):87-9.

Varicella (Chickenpox)

Summary

A mother who has chickenpox can usually provide breastmilk for her infant, but should take certain precautions in the newborn period.

Definition/cause

Varicella is a highly contagious infectious disease caused by the varicella-zoster virus, a member of the DNA containing herpesvirus family. Transmission is by direct contact of fluid from vesicles, and by airborne spread of infected respiratory droplets. In temperate climates, epidemics peak in late winter and early spring.

Among children under ten years of age, among whom the disease is most common,[1] chickenpox is usually mild and self-limiting. However, secondary cases, where the illness is acquired at home from contact, for example, with a sibling, are usually more severe than the index case, in which an older child has contracted the disease outside the home.[1]   Adolescents, adults, those on intermittent steroids or immuno-compromised persons suffer more severe disease.   One episode usually confers life-long protection.

Signs and symptoms

The incubation period is usually 14-16 days, with a range of 10-21 days.[1] The illness begins with a low grade fever, headache and malaise, typical of many viral infections, but is quickly identified as varicella by the appearance and progression of the pruritic rash. The rash begins as a small, reddish macula, progresses to a vesicle (a 'dew drop on a rose petal') and pustule, and finally to a crusted lesion. It appears first on the trunk, face, and scalp – the hairline is a favorite site – and may involve mucous membranes like the palate, pharynx, vulva, and surface of the eye.   Its distribution is central, in contrast to the distal distribution which used to be seen in smallpox.

Characteristically the rash comes in crops: the patient will have all stages of the rash and all sizes of lesions at the same time and in the same area of the body.   A classic case of varicella in a previously well child may generate 250-300 lesions;[1]   more severe cases may involve upward of 500 lesions.   Individuals are contagious for 24-48 hours preceding the onset of the rash, and until all the lesions are crusted over (about five to seven days).

Complications   include   secondary   bacterial   infections   of chickenpox   lesions   due   to   group   A   *streptococcus   pyogenes*   or *Staphylococcus aureus*.   Pneumonia can occur in adults and others at risk of more serious disease.

Treatment

Treatment is symptomatic: liquids, rest; acetaminophen to reduce pain and fever, and antipyretic therapies such as calamine lotion and oatmeal baths.   Aspirin should be avoided in children because of the risk of Reye syndrome; non steroidal anti-inflammatory drugs should also be avoided if possible, as they have been associated with worsening the disease.[1]   In newborns, anti-viral medications such as acyclovir may be used.   Children should be monitored for secondary bacterial infections.

A recently developed, live-attenuated varicella vaccine is now recommended by the American Academy of Pediatrics, to be given to all children between the ages of 12 and 18 months (in a single dose), and to teenagers who have not been vaccinated (as two doses, one to two months apart).   The varicella vaccine should not be given to children under one year of age or to pregnant women, but can be given to lactating women at high risk of exposure to the varicella-zoster virus.[1]

Varicella and breastfeeding

Varicella can be a dangerous disease if contracted during pregnancy or in the newborn period.   If a pregnant woman is infected with varicella in the first or second trimester, spontaneous abortion may occur, or the infant may be born with multiple congenital anomalies involving limbs, eyes, brain, and scarring of the skin.   If the woman becomes infected after 20 weeks of pregnancy, the fetus may get inapparent varicella – developing and recovering from the disease in utero - and then have zoster early in life without extrauterine varicella.

If a mother develops the disease five days or less before delivery and within 48 hours after delivery, the baby has been exposed to the virus in utero or at birth, within a highly susceptible window. Maternal antibodies have not had time to transfer to the neonate via the placenta, and the baby is at risk of contracting severe disease, which may be fatal.   The infant should receive varicella-zoster immune globulin (VZIG) and anti viral drugs (IV acyclovir). Because the newborn would be at increased risk of developing the disease by continued contact with a contagious mother, mother and newborn should be separated until the all her lesions are crusted over and she is no longer infectious.

Currently, it is simply not known whether the varicella virus is excreted into human milk, or whether an infant can be infected by breastfeeding.[1]   A single case report dating from 1986 found no evidence of the varicella-zoster virus in the breastmilk of two infected mothers,[2] however no recent studies have confirmed or denied this finding.   The clinician should share this fact with the parents of a newborn, who may then make an informed decision on whether or not to provide breastmilk for the neonate. If the healthy infant is exposed to the varicella-zoster virus after three weeks of age, the disease is usually mild,[3] thus continued breastfeeding is not of concern.

Food for thought
- Chickenpox is a much feared disease in hospitals. It is highly contagious, and can be widely transmitted via the ventilation system, causing problems for the many immune suppressed patients.
- The varicella-zoster virus causes primary (chickenpox), latent, and recurrent infections.   Reactivation of the latent infection causes herpes zoster (shingles).
- There are eight members of the human herpesvirus family:
    - Varicella-zoster virus
    - Herpes simplex type one (oral)
    - Herpes simplex type two (genital)
    - Cytomegalovirus
    - Epstein-Barr virus

-Human herpesvirus type 6
-Human herpesvirus type 7
-Human herpesvirus type 8

References

1. American Academy of Pediatrics.   In:Pickering LK.   ed. *2000 Red Book: Report of the Committee on Infectious Diseases.* 25th ed. Elk Grove Village, IL:American Academy of Pediatrics; 2000:624-38.
2. Frederick IB, White RJ, Braddock SW.   Excretion of varicella-herpes zoster virus in breast milk. *Am J Obstet Gynecol* 1986;154(5):1116-7.
3. Lawrence RA, Lawrence RM. *Breastfeeding: A Guide for the Medical Profession.* 5th ed. St. Louis: Mosby; 1999:585-88.

Weaning

Summary
The American Academy of Pediatrics (AAP) recommends exclusive breastfeeding for all infants until approximately six months of age, continuing to a year or beyond, with the addition of complementary solid foods at about six months.[1]

Definition/cause
Weaning is a process, common to all mammalian species, which begins when other foods besides breastmilk are offered to the infant, and ends with the cessation of breastfeeding.

Weaning and breastfeeding
In human beings, age of weaning is largely determined by cultural tradition.   Landmark work by ethnographer Clellan Ford in the 1940s surveyed reproductive and breastfeeding patterns among 64 different societies, many of them from 'primitive' cultures.   He found that many groups breastfed for three to four years, and some for as many as six years or more.   However, early introduction of solids to young infants was also common.   Ford concluded, "regardless of the availability and use of other suitable foods, weaning seems to be delayed as long as it is at all possible in the great majority of our primitive societies."[2]

Anthropologist Katherine Dettwyler studied human breastfeeding and developmental stages with suckling duration and developmental milestones in other primates.   Comparing human and primate data on age of teething, attainment of adult weight, adult body size, gestational length, and eruption of first permanent molar, she concludes, "if humans weaned their offspring according to the primate pattern, without regard to beliefs and customs, most children would be weaned between 2.5 and seven years of age."[3]

In many industrialized societies, weaning traditionally occurs far earlier than this: despite the AAP recommendations, only 21.6% of US women nurse their infants until six months of age.[4]   However, many western women do breastfeed their children into toddlerhood, and the clinician should respect each mother's goals and choices. Long-term nursing is a normal human experience, not an unusual behavior.   According to Ruth Lawrence, MD, "Unfortunately, many mothers are driven to 'closet nursing' by insensitive, uninformed relatives and friends and even physicians..... Thousands of normal, healthy children are breastfeeding until they are 3 or 4 years old.   The benefits of human milk continue."[5]

It is also important to reassure the nursing mother that normal developmental stages should not be interpreted as the infant 'rejecting' the breast.   Many infants go through a distractible phase at around five months of age, which some mothers misinterpret as a desire to wean.   When older babies learn to walk they are fascinated with this new developmental skill, and may nurse infrequently for a short period, due to their developmental stage.

Abrupt weaning

Sometimes, due to an unavoidable separation of mother and infant; a dramatic event such as an automobile accident; or an infant death, abrupt weaning is necessary.   In possibly tragic or unhappy circumstances, the mother's comfort should not be overlooked.   A fully breastfeeding woman who must suddenly stop nursing will become engorged, and unless she is experienced and efficient at hand-expression, should try to use a good quality breast pump to relieve the engorgement.

The mother should pump as necessary to prevent massive engorgement, but for as short a time as possible: if she pumps too often or for too long, she will continue to produce milk.   At first, she may need to pump approximately every four hours, for five minutes or more.   Gradually, she can lengthen the time between pumpings, and decrease the duration of each pumping, eventually discontinuing pumping entirely.   A mother experienced in hand expression may be able to achieve the same end by relieving engorgement as necessary by hand.

When an infant dies, some women find that pumping and donating milk for other sick infants helps them to cope with their loss. The mother who wants to donate milk should contact the nearest milk bank.

Deliberate weaning

Deliberate weaning occurs when the mother decides to replace breastmilk with an alternative form of nutrition.   The mother may decide to wean deliberately because of a return to work or school; because the child is starting solids, or because others are persuading her that the baby is too old to nurse.   If a mother asks for information about whether or not to wean, the clinician should be able to offer practical suggestions about continuing to breastfeed, as well as insight into weaning methods.   For example, if the mother is returning to work, an electric breast pump can help her to continue breastfeeding.

If the mother has decided that she wants to wean, deliberate weaning of an infant younger than six months of age is best achieved by gradually substituting one breastfeed at a time with a bottle of infant formula.   Similarly, in an older baby, the mother can eliminate one feed at a time, substituting as appropriate with liquid or solid foods.   As her body adjusts to each missed feed by producing less milk, the mother can eliminate another breastfeed, then another. Because the milk supply adapts, and continues to function on the principle of supply and demand, it is possible to retain, for example, the evening breastfeed, for as long as the mother wants to continue partial breastfeeding.   Often, for the sake of the child's comfort, the last feeds to go are the early morning and late evening feeds

Gradual weaning

For women who nurse long term, the issue of just how long to continue often arises: at some stage, even the most stalwart nursing mother may wonder whether her child plans to nurse into the teenage years. Breastfeeding support groups such as La Leche League (international), the Nursing Mother's Council (USA), the Nursing Mothers' Association (Australia), and the National Childbirth Trust (UK) can provide the long-term breastfeeder with practical and moral support.

Mothers with older nursing children often have questions about ending breastfeeding without distressing the child. Nursing at this stage is as often about comfort, habit, and enjoyment as it is about food. Other treats or comfort measures can substitute for nursing sessions if the mother chooses. Habitual nursing (for example, nursing every morning when the young child wakes up) may be modified by completely changing the habit: if the mother usually nurses in bed in the early morning, she can be up and dressed with breakfast ready when the child wakens. A toddler may completely forget the nursing session if the habits around it are altered.

Food for thought

- Nursing involves far more than food. Nurture is as necessary to the developing child as nourishment, and breastfeeding provides both. It is difficult to imagine any process more fundamental than weaning to a mammalian species.
- Some religions advise breastfeeding until two years of age.
- Juliet, the heroine in Shakespeare's *Romeo and Juliet*, was breastfed until age three.[6]
- Rumors maintained that Franklin D Roosevelt breastfed until he was at least three years old.[7]

Resources

The Nursing Mother's Guide to Weaning. By Kathleen Huggins and Linda Zeidrich. Harvard Common Press, US $10.95.
Mothering Your Nursing Toddler. By Norma Jane Bumgarner. La Leche League International, US $12.95.

References

1. American Academy of Pediatrics: Work Group on Breastfeeding. Breastfeeding and the Use of Human Milk. *Pediatrics* 1997;100(6):1035-1039.
2. Ford CS. *A comparative study of human reproduction.* New Haven, CT: Human Relations Area Files Press, 1964.
3. Stuart-Macadam P, Dettwyler K. *Breastfeeding: Biocultural Perspectives.* New York:Aldine de Gruyter, 1995.
4. Ryan AS. The resurgence of breastfeeding in the United States. *Pediatrics* 1997;99(4):E12.
5. Lawrence RA, Lawrence RM. *Breastfeeding: A Guide for the Medical Profession.* 5th ed. St. Louis: Mosby; 1999:346.
6. Shakespeare, W. *Romeo and Juliet.* Act I, Scene iii.
7. Cook, BW. *Eleanor Roosevelt.* Vol 1. Penguin Books, 1993:146.

Appendix

Glossary

acetylcholine	a neurotransmitter substance
acidosis	the above normal concentration of ions in the arterial blood
adenitis	inflammation of a lymph node
albumin	the main protein found in human blood
alveoli	(in lactation) milk containing sacs in the breast
amenorrhea	lack of menstruation
anastomosis	a normal route of communication between two body vessels
ankylosing spondylitis	an inflammation of the vertebra or vertebrae leading to joint stiffness
antecubital fossas	the inner part of the elbow from where blood is drawn
aqueduct of Sylvius	part of the brain
arthralgia	pain in a joint
ataxic	when an individual cannot co-ordinate muscle activity, leading to involuntary movements
autosomal recessive	an anomaly resulting from a mutation to a gene on the non-sex determining chromosome
axillary incision	a surgical incision under the arm
bacteremia	bacteria in the blood
bacteriostatic	inhibiting the growth of bacteria
bilirubin	a pigment in the blood, most of which comes from heme degradation
blepharitis	inflammation of the eyelids
bone matrix	the intercellular material of bone tissue
buccal	pertaining to the cheeks
bulla	a large blister containing fluid intestinal epithelial cells the cellular layer that lines the gut (intestines)
cellulitis	inflammation of the skin
cerebral calcifications	calcium deposits in the brain
cholangitis	inflammation of the bile duct or of multiple bile ducts
chorioamnionitis	an inflammation of the chorion, the amnion, and the amniotic fluid
circumareolar surgery	a surgical incision around the entire areola-nipple
cirrhosis	a progressive liver disease

Appendix

conjunctivitis	inflammation of the conjunctiva, the outer lining of the eye
corneal dystrophy	abnormal cornea
corticosteroids	a steroid made by the adrenal cortex
coryza	runny nose
Crigler Najjar syndrome	a defect in the liver which prevents the affected individual from processing bilirubin and can result in dangerous hyperbilirubinemia
cytochromes	a type of blood protein
cytopathy	a cellular disorder
distal	at the farthest point away from
duodenal atresia	abnormally developed section of the small intestine (in the duodenum)
dysphagia	difficulty swallowing
dysuria	painful urination
ecchymosis	purplish patches due to blood leaking into skin, like petechiae but larger
'blueberry muffin spots'	dark patches within the skin indicating blood leakage (seen with certain infections such as TORCH infections)
encephalopathy	a disorder of the brain
endocarditis	inflammation of the lining of the heart
endocervicitis	inflammation of the lining and glands of the cervix
endotracheal	inside the trachea
enterohepatic reabsorption	the reabsorption of substances in the GI tract back into the bloodstream (such as bilirubin in the newborn)
enterovirus	a virus that causes intestinal tract disease
epicanthal fold	an extra fold of skin at the corner of the eye
epidermis	the outer layer of the skin
epididymitis	an inflammation of the epididymis
erysipelas	an acute, rapidly spreading cellulitis
erythema nodosum	self-limited, recurring lesions characterized by painful nodes on the exterior surfaces of the lower extremities
erythematous	marked by redness
erythropoeisis	the creation of red blood cells
extensor surfaces of limbs	the surface of the limb exposed when the limb is extended
fine needle aspiration	a technique that involves inserting a needle into an abscess (or other such mass) and drawing out fluid
fissure	a deep slit

fistula	an abnormal passage from one body area to another
Fitz-Hugh-Curtis Syn.	perihepatitis seen with gonorrheal infection
foramina	openings through a membranous structure, such as the brain
frenotomy	a minor procedure to cut the frenulum
friable	dry or brittle
galactogogue	a substance that increases milk supply
ganglia	a cluster of nerve cells of the peripheral nervous system
giardiasis	infection with the parasite Giardia lamblia
gingivostomatitis	inflammation of the tissue inside the mouth
glaucoma	an eye disease involving increased intraocular pressure that could lead to atrophy of the optic nerve if untreated
glossitis	inflammation of the tongue
glossoptosis	irregular positioning of the tongue
glycolipids	a compound made up of a lipid and a carbohydrate
glycoproteins	a compound containing carbohydrate and protein
glomerulonephritis	inflammation of the glomerula within the kidneys
gram positive	when a stained organism takes on a blue appearance
hematocrit	the percentage of a blood sample filled by red blood cells
hematuria	the presence of blood in the urine
hemolytic anemia	anemia due to abnormal destruction of the red blood cells (such as that seen in sickle cell disease)
hepatosplenomegaly	enlargement of the liver and the spleen
hilar adenopathy	an abnormal enlargement (usually refers to the chest area)
homocysteine	an amino acid
hydrolyzed formula	a 'predigested' formula/a formula in which the components have been broken down to basic levels
hydroxylation	when the 'OH' group is added or substituted for something in a compound
hyperbilirubinemia	an excess of bilirubin in the blood
hypereflexia	increased reflexes
hyperesthesia	increased sensitivity to touch, pain or other sensory stimuli
hypernatremia	an elevated concentration of sodium in the blood

hypertrophy	enlargement of an organ or body tissue
hypoalbuminemia	low amounts of albumin in the blood
hypoperfusion	a lack of blood supply
hypoplasia	under-development of an organ or body tissue
hypoplastic	smaller than the expected size or under-development
hypoxia	below normal levels of oxygen
ileostomy	a surgically created opening which allows the ileum to discharge to the outside of the body instead of via the anus
ileum	a section of the small intestine
impetigo	a contagious, yellow-crusted skin infection
induced lactation	the creation of a milk supply in a nonpuperal woman who has not recently given birth, and who may or may not have previously been pregnant or nursed other children
infarction	insufficiency of blood supply leading to death of tissue
infrasubmammary incision	a surgical incision under the breast
interstitial pneumonitis	inflammation of the lungs within the interstitium
intubation	insertion of a hollow tube into a body canal, for example, to allow an individual to breathe, or to administer an anesthetic
in utero	within the uterus
ischemia	localized anemia due to a lack of blood flow resulting in cell death
isotonic	having an identical solute concentration as another solute concentration
lactobacillus bifidus	organisms found in the intestinal tract
lactoferrins	iron binding protein found in excretions like human milk; in the gut lactoferrin inhibits growth of organisms that depend on iron
lactogenesis	the creation of the milk supply (milk production)
lactotrophic	prolactin-producing
lateral ventricle	one of the naturally occuring spaces within the brain
lichenification	thickening of the skin
lingual frenulum	the tissue which connects the underside of the tongue to the lower part of the mouth
lumbar puncture	the insertion of a hollow needle into the subarachnoid space to obtain cerebrospinal fluid for analysis
lymphadenopathy	a disorder of the lymph nodes
lymphedema	abnormal blockage of the lymphatic vessels resulting in lymph accumulation in soft tissue

lymphogranuloma venerum	a sexually transmitted disease caused by one strain of the Chlamydia trachomatis bacterium
macula	a small flat spot on the skin
mastoiditis	inflammation of the mastoid
meconium	the black, thick, sticky stool of a newborn infant in the first one to two days of life
meningomyelocele	a ballooning out of soft tissue of meninges and the myelocele in a case of spina bifida
methionine	a nutritionally necessary amino acid
metoclopramide	a medication commonly caused to treat nausea, which can increase milk supply
microcephaly	a small head
micrognathia	an abnormally small jaw
microophthalmia	an abnormally small eye
mucocutaneous	mucous membrane and skin
mucoid	mucus-like
myalgia	muscular pain
myoglobin	the muscle protein that transports oxygen
nail dystrophy	abnormal nails
nasopharynx	the part of the throat extending from the back of the nasal opening to the soft palate
nephropathy	disorder of the kidney
neuropathy	disorder of the nervous system
nuchal	at the back of the neck
obligate anaerobe	an organism which need oxygen to live
obligate intracellular bact.	bacterial that live only when inside a cell
oculomotor	pertaining to a cranial nerveoligosaccharides a compound made up of simple sugars (monosaccharides)
opisthotonos	a spasm involving the spine and extremities
oral aphthous	an ulcerative lesion in the mouth
osteochondritis	inflammation of a bone and the surrounding cartilage
parenteral	introduction into the body which is not via the GI tract
patent ductus arteriosus	open fetal vessel that connects the left pulmonary artery to the descending aorta, which usually closes after birth
periareloar incision	a surgical incision around the entire areola
pericarditis	inflammation of the membrane which covers the heart
perihepatitis	inflammation of the covering of the liver
periorbital	around the orbit or eye socket
periostitis	inflammation of the fibrous membrane which covers the bones

petechiae	a type of rash made up of purplish pencil-tip size spots on the skin which do not blanche under pressure
pharyngeal	pertaining to the pharynx (upper portion of the digestive tract)
phenylacetic acid	a breakdown product of phenylalanine
phenylalanine	an amino acid
phenylalanine hydroxylase	an enzyme needed for the breakdown of phenylalanine
phenylketones	breakdown products of phenylalanine which, in large amounts, are harmful to the cells of the developing nervous system
phenylpyruvic acid	a breakdown product of phenylalanine
photophobia	a fear or dislike of light
pleural effusion	an accumulation of fluid in the pleural space around the lungs
polydipsia	excessive thirst
polymorphism	existence of multiple forms
polyphasia	excessive hunger, appetite, or eating
polyuria	excessive urination
popliteal fossa	the back side of the knee
preeclampsia	a condition which involves abnormally high blood pressure during the later part of pregnancy
proctitis	inflammation of the rectum
protozoa	a single-celled or non-cellular life form
pruritus	itching
psychotropes	substances which affect the mind (as in certain medications)
ptosis	the prolapse of an organ
puerperal mastitis	mastitis occurring in the postpartum period
pustule	a small, well defined elevation of the skin that contains pus
pyoderma	a pus-forming skin infection
pyoderma gangrenosum	chronic spreading of non infectious ulcers
pyruvate kinase deficiency	a disorder resulting from the lack of the enzyme pyruvate kinase
relactation	the creation of a milk supply in a woman who recently gave birth, but has not breastfed successfully, or has stopped breastfeeding
retinitis	inflammation of the retina
retinopathy	disorder of the retina
Reye's syndrome	an acquired encephalopathy usually seen in children which follows a febrile illness (often the 'flu or chickenpox), and has been associated with aspirin use in children

Appendix

rhinorrhea	nasal discharge/ a runny nose
sagital	in an anterior/posterior direction
salpingitis	inflammation of the uterine tube
sclerae	the white part of the eye
secretory IgA	an antibody secreted by the plasma cells
sepsis	the existence of bacteria or their toxins in the blood
seroconversion	the creation of antibodies in the serum in response to contact with foreign antigens
skin tag	an extra, small piece of skin
spherocytosis	a blood disorder in which red blood cells are abnormally shaped
spirochete	a type of bacteria characterized by a coiled shape
spirochetemia	the presence of spirochetes in the blood
stomatitis	inflammation of the stoma (mouth)
suppurative	pus forming
thrombocytopenia	the existence of below normal levels of platelets in the blood
total parenteral nutrition	complete nutrition, provided via an indwelling catheter into the venous circulatory system
toxic megacolon	extreme dilation of the colon
transareolar incision	a surgical incision across the areola-nipple
tyrosine	an amino acid
urethritis	an inflammation of the urethra
uveal tract	the iris, ciliary body, and choroid (of the eye)
uveitis	inflammation of the uveal tract
vesicle	a small sac or blister on the skin containing clear fluid
vesicoureteral reflux	reflux of urine from the bladder back up into the ureters or in serious cases, into the kidney
villous atrophy	villous projections which are small or wasted
viral exanthum	a rash characteristic of a particular viral illness (for example, the vesicle seen with chickenpox)
viremia	a virus in the blood

The Ten Steps to Successful Breastfeeding

1. Have a written breastfeeding policy that is routinely communicated to all health care staff.

2. Train all health care staff in skills necessary to implement this policy.

3. Inform all pregnant women about the benefits of breastfeeding.

4. Help mothers initiate breastfeeding within one hour of birth.

5. Show mothers how to breastfeed and how to maintain lactation, even if they should be separated from their infants.

6. Give newborn infants no food or drink other than breast milk, unless medically indicated.*

7. Practice rooming-in – allow mothers and infants to remain together- 24 hours a day.

8. Encourage breastfeeding on demand.

9. Give no artificial teats or pacifiers to breastfeeding infants.

10. Foster the establishment of breastfeeding support groups and refer mothers to them, on discharge from the hospital or clinic.

* A hospital must pay fair market price for all formula and infant feeding supplies that it uses, and cannot accept free or heavily discounted formula and supplies.

Web Sites for Breastfeeding Information

Academy of Breastfeeding Medicine	www.bfmed.org
Baby Friendly Hospital Initiative News	www.aboutus.com/a100/bfusa/
Baby Milk Action	www.oneworld.org/baby_milk/milk_info.html
Bestfed	www.bestfed.com
Breastfeeding	www.breastfeeding.com
Breastfeeding and Medications	http://neonatal.ttuhsc.edu/lact
Breastfeeding Legislative Updates	www.house.gov/maloney/
Breastfeeding or Nursing Mothers	www.nursingmother.com
Breastfeeding Task Force of Greater LA	www.breastfeedingtaskforla.org
Centers for Disease Control and Prevention	www.cdc.gov
Coalition to Improve Maternity Services	www.Healthy.net/CIMS/
Department of Health and Human Services	www.dhhs.gov
Food and Drug Administration	www.fda.gov
Healthy People 2010 National Objectives	http://web.heaalth.gov/HealthyPeople
Human Milk Banking Assn of North America	www.leron-line.com/milkbank.htm
International Baby Food Action Network	www.aleitamento.org.dr/ingles/ibfan.htm
International Childbirth Education Association Inc	www.icea.org
International Lactation Consultants Association	www.ilca.org
La Leche League International	www.lalecheleague.org
Promotion of Mothers Milk Inc	www.promom.org
San Diego Breastfeeding Coalition	www.breastfeeding.org
United Nations Children's Fund	www.unicef.org
WHO Code	www.tdh.texas.gov/lactate/whocode.htm#1item
World Alliance for Breastfeeding Action	www.waba.org
Breastfeeding Promotion in Pediatric office Practices	www.aap.org

Ordering Information

Pharmasoft Publishing
21 Tascocita Circle
Amarillo, Texas 79124-7301

8:00 AM to 5:00 PM CST

Sales............. 800-378-1317
806-376-9900

Fax................ 806-376-9901

Online Web Orders

http://www.iBreastfeeding.com

Single Copies $19.95 US